GENERAL SURGERY

MEDICAL STUDENT
USMLE BOARDS PARTS II AND III

PEARLS OF WISDOM

Gwenda Lyn Breckler

Kimball I. Maull

NOTE

The intent of General Surgery Medical Student Pearls of Wisdom is to serve as a study aid to improve performance on a standardized examination. It is not intended to be a source text of the knowledge base of medicine or to serve as a reference in any way for the practice of clinical medicine. Neither Boston Medical Publishing Corporation or the editors warrant that the information in this text is complete or accurate. The reader is encouraged to verify each answer in several references. All drug use indications and dosages must be verified by the reader before administration of any compound.

Copyright © 1999 by Boston Medical Publishing Corporation, Boston, MA.

Printed in U.S.A.

All rights reserved, including the right of reproduction, in whole or in part, in any form.

The editors would like to extend thanks to Terri Lair, Brad Plantz and Vicki Schlegel for their excellent managing and editorial support.

Art Director: Maryse Charette

This book was produced using Times and Symbols fonts and computer based graphics with Macintosh® computers

ISBN: 1-890369-19-5

DEDICATION

To my sister, Dorothy and my brother, Lawrence, for always beleiving in me.

Gwenda Lyn Breckler

To future physicians and surgeons — as you leave the age of innocence to enter the world of responsibility for the living and dying — may this work contribute to your making a smooth transition.

Kimball I. Maul

EDITOR IN CHIEF:

Gwenda Lyn Breckler, D.O.
Department of Surgery
Chicago Medical School
Mt. Sinai Hospital
Chicago, IL

Kimball I. Maull, M.D.
Director
The Trauma Center at Carraway
Carraway Methodist Medical Center
Birmingham, AL

CONTRIBUTING AUTHORS:

William T. Adamson, M.D.
Pediatric Surgery Fellow
The Children's Hospital of Philadelphia
Philadelphia, PA

Linda Anderson, M.D.
Department of Internal Medicine
Pulmonary and Critical Care Medicine Section
University of Nebraska Medical Center
Omaha, NE

Michael L. Ault, M.D.
Instructor in Anesthesiology
Section of Critical Care Medicine
Department of Anesthesiology
Northwestern University Medical School
Chicago, IL

Beth A. Ballinger, M.D.
Assistant professor of Vascular Surgery
The University of Iowa Hospitals and Clinics
Iowa City, IA

Dennis R. Banducci, M.D.
Associate Professor
Section of Plastic and Reconstructive Surgery
Penn State/Geisinger Health Systems
Hershey, PA

Howard Belzberg, M.D.
Los Angeles County and University of Southern California Medical Center
Los Angeles, CA

Brian Bonanni, M.D.
Duke University Medical Center
Durham, NC

Jon M. Braverman, M.D.
Denver Health Medical Center
University of Colorado School of Medicine
Denver, CO

David F. M. Brown, M.D.
Instructor in Medicine
Harvard Medical School
Massachusetts General Hospital
Boston, MA

Eduardo Castro, M.D.
Instructor in Medicine
Harvard Medical School
Massachusetts General Hospital
Boston, MA

Willie Chen, M.D.
Louisville, KY

Charles H. Cook, M.D.
Assistant Professor of Surgery and Critical Care
The Ohio State University Hospitals
Columbus, OH

Joseph T. Cooke, M.D., FACCP
Associate Professor of Clinical Medicine
Associate Director, Medical Critical Care
The New York Hospital-Cornell Medical Center
New York, NY

William M. Coplin, M.D.
Assistant Professor
Neurology and Neurological Surgery
Wayne State University
Detroit, MI

C. James Corrall, M.D., MPH
Clinical Associate Professor of Pediatrics
Clinical Associate Professor of Emergency Medicine
Indiana University School of Medicine
Indianapolis, IN

John D. Corson, M.B., Ch.B, FRCS, FACS
Department of Surgery
The University of Iowa Hospitals and Clinics
Iowa City, IA

Douglas B. Coursin, M.D.
Professor of Anesthesiology and Internal Medicine
Associate Director of the Trauma and Life Support Center
University of Wisconsin School of Medicine
Madison, WI

G. Paul Dabrowski, M.D.
Assistant Professor of Surgery
University of Pennsylvania
Philadelphia, PA

Brian J. Daley, M.D.
Assistant Professor
Division of Trauma and Critical Care
The University of Tennessee Medical Center
Knoxville, TN

Carl W. Decker, M.D.
Madigan Army Medical Center
Fort Lewis, WA

Joshua De Leon, M.D.
Assistant Professor of Medicine
Mount Sinai School of Medicine
New York, NY
Director, Cardiac Catherization and Invasive Cardiology
Elmhust Hospital Center
Elmhurst, NY

Dennis D. Diaz, M.D.
Assistant Professor of Surgery
Department of Otolaryngology-Head and Neck Surgery
Penn State/Geisinger Health Systems
Hershey, PA

Gerard M. Doherty, M.D.
Assistant Professor of Surgery
Washington University School of Medicine
St. Louis, MO

Peter Emblad, M.D.
Boston City Hospital
Boston, MA

Ron M. Fairman, M.D.
Assistant Professor of Surgery
University of Pennsylvania
Philadelphia, PA

Phillip Fairweather, M.D.
Clinical Assistant Professor
Mount Sinai School of Medicine
New York, NY
Department of Emergency Medicine
Elmhurst Hospital Center
Elmhurst, NY

Craig Feied, M.D.
Clinical Associate Professor
George Washington University
Washington Hospital Center
Washington, D.C.

Louis Flancbaum, M.D., FACS, FCCM, FCCP
Associate Professor of Surgery, Anesthesiology, and Human Nutrition
The Ohio State University Hospitals
Columbus, OH

Seth Daniel Force, M.D.
Instructor in Surgery
University of Pennsylvania
Philadelphia, PA

Mark Franklin, M.D.
Department of Anesthesiology
Northwestern University Medical School
Chicago, IL

Richard Freeman, M.D.
Section of General Thoracic Surgery
School of Medicine
University of Washington
Seattle, WA

Rajesh R. Gandhi, M.D.
Critical Care/Trauma Fellow
University of Pennsylvania
Philadelphia, PA

Judith L. Geidebring, M.D.
Lecturer
University of Michigan
Ann Arbor, MI

Robert J. Gewirtz, M.D.
Assistant Professor of Neurosurgery
Department of Surgery
University of Kentucky
Chandler Medical Center
Lexington, KY

Sheree Givre, M.D.
Clinical Assistant Professor
Department of Emergency Medicine
Mount Sinai School of Medicine
New York, NY
Associate Director
Department of Emergency Medicine
Elmhurst Hospital Center
Elmhurst, NY

John T. Gorczyca, M.D.
Assistant Professor
Division of Orthopaedic Surgery
University of Kentucky
Chandler Medical Center
Lexington, KY

Bill Gossman, M.D.
Chicago Medical School
Mt. Sinai Medical Center
Chicago, IL

Vicente H. Gracias, M.D.
Instructor of Surgery and Trauma
Surgical Critical Care Fellow
University of Pennsylvania
Philadelphia, PA

Rajan Gupta, M.D.
Instructor of Surgery and Trauma
Surgical Critical Care Fellow
University of Pennsylvania
Philadelphia, PA

Wesley Hall, M.D.
Division of Plastic and Reconstructive Surgery
Penn State/Geisinger Health System
Hershey, PA

Susan M. Harding, M.D.
Assistant Professor of Medicine
Pulmonary and Critical Care Medicine
University of Alabama
Birmingham, AL

Randy M. Hauck, M.D.
Assistant Professor of Surgery
Division of Plastic and Reconstructive Surgery
Penn State/Geisinger Health System
Hershey, PA

Marilyn T. Haupt, M.D.
Professor, Department of Medicine
Wayne State University School of Medicine
Detroit, MI

Jeffrey W. Hawkins, M.D.
Co-Director, Pulmonary and Critical Care
Medicine
Norwood Clinic
Birmingham, AL

Thomas W. Hejkal, M.D.
Department of Ophthalmology
University of Nebraska Medical Center
Omaha, NE

Timothy C. Hodges, M.D.
Assistant Professor in Surgery
School of Medicine
University of Missouri, Kansas City
Kansas City, MO

James F. Holmes, M.D.
University of California, Davis
School of Medicine
Sacramento, CA

Todd K. Howard, M.D.
Washington University
School of Medicine
St. Louis, MO

May Huang, M.D.
Assistant Professor
Neurotology & Otology
Penn State/Geisinger Health System
Hershey, PA

Charles B. Huddleston, M.D.
Washington School of Medicine
Washington University
St. Louis, MO

Karen S. Hunter, M.D.
Assistant Professor
Division of Trauma/Critical Care
The University of Tennessee
Knoxville, TN

Kamal MF Itani, M.D.
Assistant Professor
Baylor College of medicine
Associate Chief, Surgery
Chief, Ambulatory Surgery
Veterans Affairs Medical Center
Houston TX

Shyam Ivaturi, M.D.
Ridgeland, MS

Jeffrey S. Jacobs, M.D.
Assistant Professor of Anesthesiology
Miami VAMC/Jackson Memorial Hospital
University of Miami
Miami, FL

M. Salik A. Jahania, M.D.
Resident General Surgery
Post Doctoral Research Fellow
Department of Surgery
University of Kentucky College of Medicine
Lexington, KY

Cameron Javid, M.D.
Department of Ophthalmology
Tulane University
New Orleans, LA

Keith Jeffords, M.D., D.D.S.
Resident
Section of Plastic and Reconstructive Surgery
Penn State/Geisinger Health Systems
Hershey, PA

Marc J. Kahn, M.D.
Assistant Professor of Medicine
Internal Medicine Residency Program Director
Associate Director for Student Programs
Department of Medicine
Section of Hematology/Medical Oncology
Tulane University School of Medicine
New Orleans, LA

Henry J. Kaminski, M.D.
Case Western Reserve University School of Medicine
Department of Veterans Affairs Medical Center
University Hospitals of Cleveland
Cleveland, OH

Stuart Kessler, M.D.
Vice Chairman, Department of Emergency Medicine
Mount Sinai School of Medicine
New York, NY
Director, Department of Emergency Medicine
Elmhurst Hospital Center
Elmhurst, NY

Ali M. Khorrami, M.D., Ph.D.
University Eye Institute
Syracuse, NY

Albert S. Khouri, M.D.
Kentucky Lions Eye Center
Louisville, KY

Walter Koltun, M.D.
Department of Surgery
Penn State/Geisinger Health System
Hershey, PA

Lance W. Kreplick, M.D.
Assistant Professor
University of Illinois
EHS Christ Hospital
Oak Lawn, IL

Andrew Lee, M.D.
Department of Ophthalmology
Baylor College of Medicine
Houston, TX

Kevin R. Lee, M.D.
Chief Resident
Neurological Surgery
Wayne State University
Detroit, MI

Klaus-Dieter K.L. Lessnau, M.D.
New York, NY

Roger J. Levin, M.D.
Assistant Professor of Surgery
Section of Otolaryngology
Head and Neck Surgery
Penn State Geisinger Health System
Penn State University College of Medicine
Hershey, PA

Gillian Lewke, P.A., CMA
Physician Assistant
Rockford Memorial Hospital
Rockford, IL

Joseph Lieber, M.D.
Associate Attending in Medicine
Chief, Medical Consult Service
Elmhurst Hospital Center
Elmhurst, NY
Clinical Associate Professor of Medicine
Mount Sinai School of Medicine
New York, NY

Mary W. Lieh-Lai, M.D.
Director, ICU
Associate Professor, Department of Pediatrics
Children's Hospital of Michigan
Wayne State University School of Medicine
Detroit, MI

Marijana Ljubanovic, M.D.
Fellow in Critical Care Medicine
Section of Critical Care Medicine
Department of Anesthesiology
Northwestern University Medical School
Chicago, IL

Walter Longo, M.D.
St. Louis University Medical Center
St. Louis, MO

Bernard Lopez, M.D.
Assistant Professor
Thomas Jefferson Medical College
Thomas Jefferson University Hospital
Philadelphia, PA

John T. Malcynski, M.D.
Instructor of Surgery and Trauma
Surgical Critical Care Fellow
University of Pennsylvania
Philadelphia, PA

Lloyd Maliner, M.D.
Section of Neurosurgery
Penn State Geisinger Health System
Hershey, PA

Sanjeev Maniar, M.D.
Department of Neurology
Wayne State University
Detroit, MI

Gregory P. Marelich, M.D., FACP, FCCP
Assistant Professor of Clinical Internal
Medicine
Division of Pulmonary and Critical Care
Medicine
University of California Davis Medical Center
Sacramento, CA

Robert G. Martindale, M.D., Ph.D.
Associate Professor of Surgery
Section of Gastrointestinal Surgery
Medical College of Georgia
Augusta, GA

Joseph Masci, M.D.
Associate Director of Medicine
Mount Sinai Services
Elmhurst Hospital Center
Elmhurst, NY
Associate Professor of Medicine
Mount Sinai School of Medicine
New York, NY

Terence McGarry, M.D.
Pulmonary and Critical Care Medicine
Elmhurst Hospital Center
Elmhurst, NY
Assistant Professor of Medicine
Mount Sinai School of Medicine
New York, NY

Luis Mejico, M.D.
Department of Neurology
Georgetown University Medical Center
Washington, DC

Eric N. Mendeloff, M.D.
Assistant Professor of Surgery
Washington School of Medicine
Washington University
St. Louis, MO

Kevin Miller, M.D.
Jules Stein Eye Institute
Los Angeles, CA

Ravi Moonka, M.D.
Staff Surgeon
Puget Sound Veterans Affairs Medical Center
Clinical Instructor
Department of Surgery
University of Washington Medical Center
Seattle, WA

Gholam K. Motamedi, M.D.
Department of Neurology
Baylor College of Medicine
Houston, TX

Debasish Mridha, M.D.
Resident (PGY-4)
Department of Neurology
Wayne State University School of Medicine
Detroit, MI

Anthony M. Murro, M.D.
Associate Professor of Neurology
Department of Neurology
Medical College of Georgia
Augusta, GA

Debra Myers, M.D.
Pulmonary/Critical Care Division
Sleep Disorders Medicine
Assistant Professor
Department of Internal Medicine
Wayne State University School of Medicine
Detroit, MI

Michael L. Nance, M.D.
Schnaufer Senior Surgical Fellow
The Children's Hospital of Philadelphia
Philadelphia, PA

Prashant K. Narain, M.D.
Department of Surgery
Medical College of Virginia
Richmond, VA

Munier Nazzal, M.D., FRCS
Department of Surgery
The University of Iowa Hospitals and Clinics
Iowa City, IA

Kurt M. Nellhaus, M.D., FCCP
Pulmonary Service, Department of Medicine
Lakes Region General Hospital
Laconia, NH

David Neschis, M.D.
Department of Surgery
University of Pennsylvania
Philadelphia, PA

Juan B. Ochoa, M.D.
Assistant Professor of General Surgery
Section of Trauma and Critical Care
University of Kentucky
Lexington, KY

Scott Olitsky, M.D.
Children's Hospital of Buffalo
Buffalo, NY

Lavi Oud, M.D.
Department of Critical Care Medicine
Wayne State University School of Medicine
Detroit, MI

Carlos A. Pellegrini, M.D.
Professor and Chairman
Department of Surgery
University of Washington Medical Center
Seattle, WA

Thomas J. Poulton, M.D., FACP, FAAP, FCCM, FCCP
Professor and Chairman
Department of Anesthesiology
Fletcher Allen Health Care
University of Vermont College of Medicine
Burlington, VT

Stephen K. Powers, M.D.
Professor and Chief
Section of Neurosurgery
Penn State Geisinger Health System
Hershey, PA

Anthony T. Reder, M.D.
Associate Professor of Neurology
Department of Neurology
The University of Chicago
Chicago, IL

Laurie Reeder, M.D.
Section of General Thoracic Surgery
School of Medicine
University of Washington
Seattle, WA

Juan Carlos Restrepo, M.D.
Diplomat of the American Board of Anesthesiology
Board Certified in Critical Care Medicine
VA Medical Center – Jackson Memorial Hospital
University of Miami
Miami, FL

Lisa Rogers, D.O.
Associate Professor of Neurology
Wayne State University School of Medicine
Detroit, MI

Carlo Rosen, M.D.
Instructor in Medicine
Harvard Medical School
Massachusetts General Hospital
Boston, MA

Jeffrey Rosenfeld, Ph.D., M.D.
Director Neuromuscular Program
Carolinas Medical Center-Internal Medicine
Charlotte, NC

David Rubenstein, M.D.
Division of Cardiology
Elmhurst Hospital Center
Elmhurst, NY

Robert L. Ruff, M.D., Ph.D.
Departments of Neurology and Neurosciences
Case Western Reserve University School of Medicine
Department of Veterans Affairs Medical Center
University Hospitals of Cleveland
Cleveland, OH

Nelson R. Sabates, M.D.
Eye Foundation of Kansas City
University of Missouri, Kansas City School of Medicine
Kansas City, MO

Juan A. Sanchez, M.D.
Assistant Professor
Department of Surgery
University of Kentucky College of Medicine
Lexington, KY

Jeannie F. Savas, M.D.
Department of Surgery
Medical College of Virginia
Richmond, VA

William B. Schroder, M.D.
Chief, Section of Vascular Surgery
School of Medicine
University of Missouri, Kansas City
Kansas City, MO

Anthony J. Senagore, M.D.
Associate Professor of Surgery
Interim Program Director
General Surgery Residency
Butterworth Hospital
Michigan State University
Grand Rapids, MI

Harvey M. Shanies, Ph.D., M.D.
Clinical Associate Professor of Medicine
Mount Sinai School of Medicine
New York, NY
Associate Director of Medicine for Clinical and Academic Pulmonary and Critical Care Medicine
Elmhurst Hospital Center
Elmhurst, NY

Andrew Shapiro, M.D.
Department of Surgery
Penn State Geisinger Health System
Hershey, PA

Girish D. Sharma, M.D., FCCP
Assistant Professor of Pediatrics
Section of Pediatric Pulmonology
The University of Chicago Children's Hospital
Chicago, IL

Carla Siegfried, M.D.
Department of Ophthalmology and Visual Sciences
Washington University
St. Louis, MO

Anders A.F. Sima, M.D., Ph.D.
Professor of Pathology and Neurology
Wayne State University School of Medicine
Detroit, MI
Visiting Professor of Pathology
University of Michigan
Ann Arbor, MI
Staff Neuropathologist
Harper Hospital and Detroit Medical Center
Detroit, MI

Sabine Sobek, M.D.
Department of Critical Care Medicine
Wayne State University School of Medicine
Detroit, MI

Dana Stearns, M.D.
Instructor in Medicine
Harvard Medical School
Massachusetts General Hospital

Jack Stump, M.D.
Attending Physician
Rogue Valley Medical Center
Medford, OR

Joan Surdukowski, M.D.
Assistant Professor
Chicago Medical School
Mt. Sinai Hospital
Chicago, IL

Michael J. Taravella, M.D.
University of Colorado
Denver, CO

William O. Tatum, IV, M.D.
Clinical Assistant Professor
Tampa General Hospital Epilepsy Center
Tampa, FL

Menno Terriet, M.D.
Department of Anesthesia
Veterans Affairs Medical Center
Miami, FL

Carlo Tornatore, M.D.
Assistant Professor of Neurology
Department of Neurology
Georgetown University Medical Center
Washington, DC

R. Scott Turner, M.D., Ph.D.
Assistant Professor Department of Neurology
University of Michigan
Ann Arbor, MI

Eric Vallieres, M.D.
Section of General Thoracic Surgery
School of Medicine
University of Washington
Seattle, WA

Mythili Venkataraman, M.D.
Attending, Pulmonary Medicine
Director, Bronchology and Invasive Procedures
Elmhurst Hospital Center
Elmhurst, NY
Assistant Professor of Medicine
Mount Sinai School of Medicine
New York, NY

Mladen Vidovich, M.D.
Department of Anesthesiology
Northwestern University Medical School
Chicago, IL

Boris Vinogradski, M.D.
Surgical Resident
Section of Trauma and Critical Care
University of Kentucky
Lexington, KY

Martin Warshawsky, M.D., FACP, FCCP
Director, Respiratory Intensive Care Unit
Elmhurst Hospital Center
Elmhurst, NY
Assistant Professor of Medicine
Mount Sinai School of Medicine
New York, NY

Kenneth E. Wood, D.O.
Assistant Professor of Medicine
Director of the Trauma and Life Support Center
University of Wisconsin School of Medicine
Madison, WI

John H. Yim, M.D.
Resident in General Surgery
Washington University School of Medicine
St. Louis, MO

Kristin Zeller, M.D.
Norfolk, VA

WE APPRECIATE YOUR COMMENTS!

We appreciate your opinion and encourage you to send us any suggestions or recommendations. Please let us know if you discover any errors, or if there is any way we can make Pearls of Wisdom more helpful to you. We are also interested in recruiting new authors and editors. Please call, write, fax, or e-mail. We look forward to hearing from you.

Return to:

Boston Medical Publishing Corporation
237 S. 70th Street, Suite 206, Lincoln, NE, 68510

888-MBOARDS (626-2737)
402-484-6118
Fax: 402-484-6552
E-mail: bmp@emedicine.com
www.emedicine.com

INTRODUCTION

Congratulations! General Surgery Medical Student Pearls of Wisdom will help you improve your knowledge base in surgery. Originally designed as a study aid to improve performance on the USMLE Surgery Board exam, Pearls is full of useful information. A few words are appropriate in discussing intent, format, limitations and use.

Since Pearls is primarily intended as a study aid, the text is written in a rapid-fire question/answer format. This way, readers receive immediate gratification. Moreover, misleading or confusing "foils" are not provided. This eliminates the risk of erroneously assimilating an incorrect piece of information that makes a big impression. The questions, themselves, often contain a "pearl" intended to reinforce the answer. Additional "hooks" may be attached to the answer in various forms, including mnemonics, visual imagery, repetition and humor. Additional information, not requested in the question, may be included in the answer. Emphasis has been placed on distilling trivia and key facts that are easily overlooked, quickly forgotten and that somehow seem to be needed on board examinations.

Many questions have answers without explanations. This enhances ease of reading and rate of learning. Explanations often occur in a later question/answer. Upon reading an answer, the reader may think, "Hm, why is that?" or "Are you sure?" If this happens to you, go check! Truly assimilating these disparate facts into a framework of knowledge absolutely requires further reading of the surrounding concepts. Information learned in response to seeking an answer to a particular question is retained much better than information that is passively observed. Take advantage of this! Use Pearls with your preferred texts handy and open.

Pearls has limitations. We have found many conflicts between sources of information. We have tried to verify in several references the most accurate information. Some texts have internal discrepancies further confounding clarification.

Pearls risks accuracy by aggressively pruning complex concepts down to the simplest kernel—the dynamic knowledge base and clinical practice of medicine is not like that! Furthermore, new research and practice occasionally deviates from that which likely represents the right answer for test purposes. This text is designed to maximize your score on a test. Refer to your most current sources of information and mentors for direction for practice.

Pearls is designed to be used, not just read. It is an interactive text. Use a 3 x 5 card and cover the answers; attempt all questions. A study method we recommend is oral, group study, preferably over an extended meal or pitchers. The mechanics of this method are simple and no one ever appears stupid. One person holds Pearls, with answers covered and reads the question. Each person, including the reader, says "Check!" when he or she has an answer in mind. After everyone has "checked" in, someone states his/her answer. If this answer is correct, on to the next one; if not, another person says their answer or the answer can be read. Usually the person who "checks" in first receives the first shot at stating the answer. If this person is being a smarty-pants answer-hog, then others can take turns. Try it, it's almost fun!

Pearls is also designed to be re-used several times to allow, dare we use the word, memorization. Two check boxes are provided for any scheme of keeping track of questions answered correctly or incorrectly. We welcome your comments, suggestions and criticism. Great effort has been made to verify these questions and answers. Some answers may not be the answer you would prefer. Most often this is attributable to variance between original sources. Please make us aware of any errors you find. We hope to make continuous improvements and would greatly appreciate any input with regard to format, organization, content, presentation or about specific questions. We also are interested in recruiting new contributing authors and publishing new textbooks. Contact our manager at Boston Medical Publishing, Terri Lair, at (toll free) 1-888-MBOARDS. We look forward to hearing from you!

Study hard and good luck!

G.L.B. & K.I.M.

TABLE OF CONTENTS

GENERAL PRINCIPLES PEARLS 15

WOUND HEALING AND NUTRITION PEARLS... 19

ANESTHESIA PEARLS.. 27

CRITICAL CARE, SHOCK, FLUIDS AND ELECTROLYTE PEARLS 34

HEENT PEARLS 52

ESOPHAGUS, STOMACH, DUODENUM AND DIAPHRAGM PEARLS 66

APPENDIX AND INGUINAL HERNIA PEARLS... 79

CARDIAC SURGERY PEARLS 84

VASCULAR SURGERY PEARLS 92

CHEST WALL, LUNG, PLEURA AND MEDIASTINUM PEARLS..........................101

LIVER, GALLBLADDER, PANCREAS AND SPLEEN PEARLS..............................109

SMALL INTESTINE, COLON, RECTUM AND ANUS PEARLS...............................126

INTRAABDOMINAL INFECTIONS AND SURGICAL COMPLICATIONS PEARLS.....................139

ABDOMINAL WALL, OMENTUM, MESENTARY AND RETROPERITONEUM PEARLS............144

ADRENAL, PITUITARY AND HYPOTHALAMUS PEARLS....................................148

THYROID AND PARATHYROID PEARLS..158

TRAUMA AND BURN PEARLS 164

ORTHOPEDIC AND HAND SURGERY PEARLS..175

BREAST SURGERY PEARLS 183

PLASTIC AND RECONSTRUCTIVE SURGERY PEARLS...187

NEUROSURGERY PEARLS...192

GENITOURINARY SURGERY PEARLS 206

PEDIATRIC SURGERY PEARLS...213

GYNECOLOGIC SURGERY PEARLS..221

HEMATOLOGY AND ONCOLOGY PEARLS..231

IMMUNOLOGY AND TRANSPLANTATION PEARLS 237

AMPUTATION PEARLS 250

BIBLIOGRAPHY...253

GENERAL PRINCIPLES PEARLS

The feasibility of an operation is not the best indication for its performance.
Henry, Lord of Birkenhead

❏❏ **What is considered a contaminated wound?**

Open traumatic wounds, gross spillage from the gastrointestinal tract, entrance into the genitourinary or biliary tract in the presence of infected urine or bile, a major break in technique and incisions in which acute inflammation is present.

❏❏ **What are the acute complications of diabetes mellitus (DM)?**

Susceptibility to infection and metabolic derangements.

❏❏ **What drugs increase the serum level of phenytoin?**

Warfarin, isoniazid, chloramphenicol, sulfonamides, disulfram, aspirin and cimetidine.

❏❏ **What is the treatment of choice for methicillin-resistant S. aureus (MRSA)?**

Vancomycin.

❏❏ **T/F: Sterilization kills all microorganisms.**

True.

❏❏ **What is the proper tetanus prophylaxis for a 5 year old child not previously immunized but who has no wound?**

A series of 4 injections of tetanus toxoid.

❏❏ **What is the strongest independent risk factor for peripheral vascular disease (PVD) of the lower extremities?**

Smoking.

❏❏ **What is the most common electrolyte abnormality seen in patients with Conn's disease?**

Hypokalemia.

❏❏ **What diastolic blood pressure typically causes postponement of elective procedures?**

110 mm Hg.

❏❏ **What clinical signs of congestive heart failure (CHF) are predictive of postoperative pulmonary edema and worsened heart failure?**

Jugular venous distention, an S3 heart sound and rales.

❏❏ **What is the most common cardiac valvular lesion found in the preoperative work-up of noncardiac patients?**

Aortic stenosis.

❏❏ **T/F: All patients with Von Willebrand's (VW) disease should receive preoperative desmopressin (DDAVP).**

False.

❏❏ **What operations are considered high cardiac risks?**

Emergent procedures, major vascular surgery, peripheral vascular surgery and prolonged procedures with significant fluid shifts or blood loss.

❏❏ **What are the indications for preoperative serum glucose evaluation?**

DM, history of steroid use and patients with a history of pancreatic, hypothalamic or adrenal disease.

❏❏ **What factors are associated with increased perioperative pulmonary complications?**

Increased age, obesity, smoking, poor nutritional status, upper respiratory tract infection (URI), type of surgical incision, duration of anesthesia and the general health of the patient.

❏❏ **What percentage of patients requiring an amputation of the lower extremity are diabetic?**

60%.

❏❏ **What are the indications for perioperative evaluation of the coagulation system?**

Liver disease, malnutrition, malabsorption, history of anticoagulant therapy, recent history of active bleeding and inability to provide a history.

❏❏ **What is the absorption rate of plain catgut?**

Ten days.

❏❏ **What risk factors determine the severity of aspiration pneumonia?**

A pH less than 2.5 and a gastric volume of 20 to 25 cc for an average adult or .04 ml/kg for children.

❏❏ **Iodophores are effective against which organisms?**

Gram-positive and gram-negative bacteria.

❏❏ **What are the indications for preoperative chest x-rays?**

Signs and symptoms of active chest disease, intrathoracic surgical procedures and patients older than 70 years who are having major surgery.

❏❏ **What is the greatest source of contamination in the operative site?**

The operative environment, which includes nonscrubbed personnel and the air over the surgical wound.

❏❏ **What is considered adequate autoclave sterilization of surgical instruments?**

30 minutes of exposure to saturated steam at a pressure of 15 to 17 psi and at a temperature of 250° F.

❏❏ **What is meant by flash autoclaving and what instruments can be safely treated in this manner?**

Flash autoclaving is applicable only to naked, unhinged instruments and involves a higher temperature (270° F) and less time (3 minutes).

☐☐ **What is the primary source of perioperative infections?**

The patient.

☐☐ **What factors predispose to postoperative dehydration?**

Preoperative deprivation of fluid, intraoperative insensible fluid losses, third-space fluid shifts and decreased postoperative fluid intake.

☐☐ **What inappropriate surgical techniques decrease the number of bacteria required to create a suppurative wound?**

Incomplete hemostasis, retained blood clots, necrotic or traumatized tissue and foreign bodies.

☐☐ **What is the foundation upon which all other antiseptic techniques rest?**

Maintenance or re-establishment of normal physiology.

☐☐ **What pathophysiologic conditions weaken a patient's local and systemic antibacterial mechanisms?**

A low cardiac output (CO), systemic hypoperfusion, respiratory insufficiency, dehydration and electrolyte imbalances.

☐☐ **Iodine has antimicrobial activity against what organisms?**

Fungi, viruses and gram-positive and gram-negative bacteria.

☐☐ **T/F: Iodophores and hexachlorophene can be used in surgical wounds.**

False.

☐☐ **What is the most effective way to decrease the number of bacteria in a heavily contaminated wound?**

High-pressure irrigation (19-gauge needle, 35 ml syringe and a sterile electrolyte solution).

☐☐ **What type of surgical gown is associated with the lowest rate of bacterial contamination?**

Plastic gowns.

☐☐ **What is the single most important factor in the management of contaminated wounds?**

Debridement of devitalized tissue.

☐☐ **What is the best way to determine the viability of muscle tissue?**

Contraction upon stimulation (not color).

☐☐ **T/F: Shoe covers decrease the risk of infection.**

False.

☐☐ **What types of wounds are considered contaminated?**

Traumatic wounds with retained devitalized tissue, foreign bodies, fecal contamination or delayed treatment, a perforated viscus and acute bacterial inflammation with purulence.

❏❏ **What patient related factors increase the risk of infection?**

Increased age, obesity, diabetes, cirrhosis, uremia, connective tissue disorders and immune deficiency states.

❏❏ **What is the disadvantage of using Dexon or vicryl sutures?**

They are braided sutures. Bacteria may be carried into the interstices and escape phagocytosis, resulting in chronic suture infection, granulomas and sinuses.

❏❏ **Why are penrose drains brought out of the abdominal cavity through a stab wound separate from the surgical incision?**

To decrease the risk of a ventral hernia and wound infection.

❏❏ **When should a severely contaminated wound be closed?**

Not until at least 4 days after injury.

❏❏ **What is the function of a wound dressing?**

To protect wounds from mechanical trauma, bacterial invasion and absorb exudate.

❏❏ **How does immobilization decrease the spread of wound microflora?**

By decreasing lymphatic flow.

❏❏ **When should perioperative antibiotic prophylaxis be initiated?**

2 hours prior to the start of surgery.

❏❏ **T/F: Chromic catgut sutures evoke a greater inflammatory reaction than plain catgut sutures.**

False.

❏❏ **When are polyglycolic acid (Dexon) sutures absorbed?**

60 to 90 days postoperatively.

❏❏ **T/F: Perioperative heparin decreases the incidence of pulmonary embolism.**

True.

❏❏ **What organism is most frequently isolated from anaerobic wound infections?**

Bacteroides species.

WOUND HEALING AND NUTRITION PEARLS

Oh, powerful bacillus, with wonder how you fill us . . . .
William T. Helmuth

❑❑ **What is the major type of collagen in tendons?**

Type I.

❑❑ **Which amino acid is unique to collagen?**

Hydroxyproline.

❑❑ **What is the function of transforming growth factor-beta (TGF-beta)?**

It stimulates growth of fibroblasts and inhibits growth of epithelial cells.

❑❑ **T/F: Bowel sounds are a good index of small bowel motility.**

False.

❑❑ **What are the major contraindications to nasoesophageal or gastric tube feedings?**

Unconsciousness and absence of laryngeal reflexes.

❑❑ **What is the caloric content of one gram of protein?**

4.0 kcal.

❑❑ **What is the most reliable and readily available method to determine an individual's caloric needs?**

Indirect calorimetry.

❑❑ **How does skin testing determine nutritional status?**

By injecting a skin antigen such as candida, the nutritional status can be indirectly measured as a function of immunocompetence. Anergy indicates malnutrition.

❑❑ **T/F: Harris-Benedict equations frequently overestimate the caloric requirements of hospitalized patients.**

True.

❑❑ **What are the components of an elemental diet?**

Monomeric or short-chain hydrolyzed protein.

❑❑ **What percentage of nonprotein caloric needs supplied by total parenteral nutrition (TPN) should be as fat?**

25%.

❑❑ **Which preoperative patients would benefit from TPN?**

Patients who undergo major surgery that would result in 10 or more days without oral intake, those with fistulas or hyperemesis and malnourished patients undergoing major surgery.

❑❑ **What is the role of glutamine in TPN or enteral solutions?**

Glutamine is a nonessential amino acid that carries ammonia. At times of stress, it may become an essential amino acid. There is some evidence to suggest that the addition of glutamine in TPN or enteral formulations may increase nitrogen balance.

❑❑ **T/F: Lipids can be given through a peripheral vein.**

True. They are isosmotic, unlike the concentrated dextrose solutions that should only be infused centrally.

❑❑ **T/F: Overfeeding can result in difficulty in weaning a patient from mechanical ventilation.**

True. This is related to increased energy expenditure, O_2 consumption and CO_2 production with a resultant increase in respiratory rate and minute ventilation.

❑❑ **T/F: It is not recommended to place patients on enteral and parenteral feedings simultaneously.**

False. On the contrary, a small amount of nutrition delivered enterally may be all that is required to gain the positive effects of this route while the parenteral route supplies the balance of caloric and protein needs.

❑❑ **A 60 year old female is taken to the operating room with TPN infusing. The solution is made up of essential amino acids and hypertonic dextrose. What is the most likely reason this solution was chosen?**

Acute renal failure (ARF).

❑❑ **When TPN is prescribed, what anions are generally used to form sodium and potassium salts?**

Chloride and acetate.

❑❑ **What laboratory findings are important for an accurate nutritional assessment?**

Absolute lymphocyte count, creatinine, albumin, total protein, transferrin, prealbumin, retinal-binding globulin, vitamin levels and skin tests.

❑❑ **What is the half-life of albumin?**

20 days. Thus, a decrease in albumin levels denotes long-term malnutrition (at least several weeks).

❑❑ **What factors can decrease retinal-binding globulin levels?**

Hyperthyroidism, liver disease, vitamin A and zinc deficiency.

❑❑ **What are the characteristics of zinc deficiency?**

Perioral rash, hair loss and poor wound healing.

❏❏ **What is the optimal calorie-to-nitrogen ratio for critically ill patients?**

100:1 to 200:1.

❏❏ **A previously healthy, well nourished, non-stressed 38 year old man requires parenteral nutrition. What is his protein requirement?**

Between 0.8 and 1.0 g/kg.

❏❏ **What is the most common severe complication of enteral nutrition?**

Aspiration.

❏❏ **T/F: All dietary carbohydrates are hydrolyzed to glucose before intestinal absorption.**

False.

❏❏ **What metabolic disease is associated with long-term TPN?**

Metabolic bone disease.

❏❏ **What are the essential fatty acids in humans?**

Linoleic and linolenic acid.

❏❏ **What metallic nutrient may require supplementation in patients on long-term TPN because it is not part of the multi-trace elements?**

Iron.

❏❏ **An order is placed for multivitamins as MVI-12. What vitamin is excluded and must be added separately to TPN solutions?**

Vitamin K.

❏❏ **When does the proliferative phase (fibroblastic phase) of wound healing usually begin?**

About the third or fourth day after injury.

❏❏ **What is tensile strength?**

The strength per unit area of tissue.

❏❏ **What type of bond holds the alpha chains of collagen to one another?**

Hydrogen bonds.

❏❏ **Where does collagen cross-linking occur?**

In the extracellular cytoplasm.

❏❏ **T/F: Healed wounds are as strong as unwounded tissue.**

False.

❏❏ **What are the most important effects of prostacyclin (PGI_2)?**

It is antagonistic to thromboxane A2 and it promotes blood flow by stimulating vasodilatation and decreasing platelet aggregation. It is thought to control tissue plasminogen activator (tPA) release.

☐☐ **What is the obligate energy source for red blood cells?**

Glucose.

☐☐ **What is peripheral parenteral nutrition (PPN)?**

PPN provides nutritional support using peripheral veins. These solutions typically contain less concentrated amino acid solutions and dilute glucose and lipid solutions.

☐☐ **What is the maximum osmolarity of solutions that should be infused into a peripheral vein?**

900 mOsm. Parenteral nutrition solutions are commonly greater than 1500 mOsm and require central venous access for delivery.

☐☐ **How long does the body's reserve of carbohydrates last during starvation?**

Glycogen stores are consumed within 24 hours.

☐☐ **Does the metabolic rate increase or decrease during starvation in a healthy subject?**

It decreases.

☐☐ **What are the goals of TPN in critically ill patients?**

To provide maintenance levels of substrates, reduce negative protein balance, stimulate protein synthesis, avoid complications and improve outcome.

☐☐ **What are the characteristics of copper deficiency?**

Anemia and neutropenia.

☐☐ **What is total energy expenditure (TEE)?**

The amount of calories burned by an individual in a 24 hour period. It is the sum of the basal metabolic rate, activity related energy expenditure, illness related energy expenditure and the thermogenic effect of feeding.

☐☐ **What are the characteristics of marasmus (simple starvation)?**

Deficiencies of lean body mass, fat and visceral protein.

☐☐ **T/F: Doses of vitamin C greater than physiologic levels improve wound healing.**

False.

☐☐ **Which amino acid is a key fuel for rapidly dividing cells?**

Glutamine.

☐☐ **What hormones are influenced by the body's response to injury?**

Plasma catecholamines, aldosterone, antidiuretic hormone, glucagon, cortisol and growth hormone.

☐☐ **What cells produce TNF?**

Macrophages.

❑❑ **What are the most important effects of leukotrienes?**

Activation of neutrophil oxidative activity and chemotaxis, stimulation of IL-1 production, myelopoiesis, increased endothelial adhesion, increased microvascular permeability and vasoconstriction.

❑❑ **How does the change in resting energy expenditure (REE) differ in the critically ill patient versus the non-stressed starving person?**

REE increases during acute illness and decreases during non-stressed starvation.

❑❑ **What is the respiratory quotient (RQ)?**

The ratio of carbon dioxide produced to oxygen consumed. When carbohydrate is the fuel, the RQ is 1.0, for protein it is 0.8 and for fat it is 0.7.

❑❑ **What does an RQ greater than 1.0 indicate?**

Fat synthesis.

❑❑ **What are the main organs involved in glucose production during starvation?**

The liver and kidney.

❑❑ **What group of patients has been shown to benefit from preoperative TPN?**

Those with severe malnutrition having major surgery.

❑❑ **What are the available concentrations of amino acid solutions for TPN in adults?**

8.5, 10 and 15%.

❑❑ **Resolution of hepatic encephalopathy may be effected by administration of parenteral formulas rich in what compounds?**

Branched-chain amino acids.

❑❑ **Lipid emulsions come in what two concentrations?**

10 and 20%.

❑❑ **What is the maximum dextrose concentration available for use in TPN?**

70% dextrose (D70). This provides 700 grams of dextrose per liter.

❑❑ **What is the maximum rate of glucose utilization?**

7 g/kg/day or 5 mg/kg/min.

❑❑ **T/F: Denervation has no effect on wound contraction or epithelialization.**

True.

❑❑ **T/F: TGF-alpha stimulates endothelial cell proliferation.**

True.

❑❑ **The first phase of metabolic and endocrine events following trauma is the catabolic (adrenergic/corticoid) phase. What does this phase involve?**

This occurs when metabolic demands and urinary excretion of nitrogen increase beyond levels associated with simple starvation. There is an obligatory mobilization of protein in an attempt to provide energy for gluconeogenesis.

❑❑ **How much carbohydrate, protein and lipid are in one liter of the following TPN prescription: AA 4 + D20 + Lip. 6.3?**

40 grams of amino acids, 200 gram of dextrose and 63 grams of fat.

❑❑ **Protein requirements are often stated in terms of nitrogen requirement. How is the content of nitrogen in dietary protein determined?**

Grams of dietary protein divided by 6.25 approximates grams of nitrogen.

❑❑ **What are the indications for tube feeding via the jejunal route?**

Comatose patients, patients without a laryngeal reflex and those in whom nasoesophageal, nasogastric or nasojejunostomy tubes cannot be placed.

❑❑ **During acute illness, what do changes in body weight reflect?**

Fluid shifts.

❑❑ **During which phase of the cell cycle do vascular endothelial cells divide?**

G1.

❑❑ **What is the composition of granulation tissue?**

New capillaries, proliferating fibroblasts and an immature matrix of collagen, proteoglycans, substrate adhesion molecules and acute and chronic inflammatory cells.

❑❑ **What is meant by negative nitrogen balance?**

The amount of nitrogen taken in by the patient is exceeded by the amount lost.

❑❑ **What is the role of chromium in human metabolism?**

Chromium promotes insulin action in peripheral tissues.

❑❑ **T/F: When a normally healing wound is disrupted after 5 days and then re-closed, the return of wound strength is more rapid than in primary healing.**

True.

❑❑ **What is the process whereby keratinocytes migrate and then divide to resurface partial-thickness skin loss?**

Epithelialization.

❑❑ **What is the primary cell that regulates collagen synthesis?**

The macrophage.

❑❑ **What is the role of fibroblasts in wound healing?**

They produce the extracellular matrix and polysaccharide gel into which the matrix is embedded.

❏❏ **In normally healing wounds, when does the maturation phase start?**

3 weeks after injury.

❏❏ **T/F: The strength of a healed wound eventually equals that of unwounded tissue.**

False.

❏❏ **What are the processes (in order) of wound healing?**

Inflammation, epithelialization, collagen synthesis and contraction.

❏❏ **What is burst strength?**

The force required to break a wound (independent of area).

❏❏ **T/F: Older individuals have less contraction and deformity of facial wounds.**

True.

❏❏ **What is the function of interferon (IFN)?**

It inhibits fibroblast proliferation and collagen synthesis.

❏❏ **What is the average resting energy consumption for a 70 kg male?**

1,500 kcal/day.

❏❏ **T/F: Vitamin A accelerates wound healing.**

False.

❏❏ **Where are branched-chain amino acids primarily metabolized?**

In the liver.

❏❏ **What percentage of dietary protein is converted to urea?**

60%.

❏❏ **T/F: Glutamine is preferentially metabolized by the liver.**

False.

❏❏ **T/F: The Krebs cycle occurs in the Golgi complex.**

False.

❏❏ **Which cell type is the primary force driving wound contraction?**

The fibroblast.

❏❏ **T/F: Older people heal more slowly.**

True.

❏❏ **What is the predominant cell type in the first 24 hours of the inflammatory phase of wound healing?**

Polymorphonuclear leukocytes (PMNs), followed by a preponderance of macrophages.

❏❏ **When has collagen synthesis reached its peak?**

5 to 7 days after injury.

❏❏ **What is the function of fibroblast growth factor (FGF)?**

It induces angiogenesis, increases epithelial cell migration and hastens wound contraction.

❏❏ **What cells produce interferon (IFN)?**

Lymphocytes and fibroblasts.

❏❏ **Which body tissue heals without scar formation?**

Bone.

❏❏ **What is the major component of the extracellular matrix?**

Collagen.

❏❏ **Which glycosaminoglycan is not sulfated or bound to protein?**

Hyaluronic acid.

❏❏ **When do fibroblasts appear in the wound?**

About the third day.

❏❏ **How long does it take for a watertight seal to form in surgical incisions?**

About 24 hours.

ANESTHESIA PEARLS

Mr. Anesthetist, if the patient can keep awake, surely you can.
Wilfred Trotter

❑❑ T/F: Nondepolarizing muscle relaxants have a short duration of action.

True.

❑❑ What is the estimated mortality due to anesthesia alone?

As low as 1:100,000 (less for healthy patients).

❑❑ During induction of general anesthesia, what happens to the diaphragm?

It shifts cephalad in the supine patient. This accounts for a loss of 340 to 750 cc of lung volume.

❑❑ How do intravenous anesthetics affect the respiratory muscles?

They depress diaphragmatic tonic activity.

❑❑ How is induction of anesthesia associated with hypoxia?

It is associated with increased dead space ventilation, shunting of blood and inhibition of hypoxic vasoconstriction.

❑❑ What is the mechanism of shunting?

Loss of normal respiratory muscle support of the lung and subsequent atelectasis.

❑❑ What is absorption atelectasis?

Atelectasis that occurs when 100% oxygen is administered. Without the presence of slowly diffusing nitrogen, the oxygen is completely absorbed from the airspaces.

❑❑ What are the advantages of ambulatory pediatric anesthesia?

Reduction of cost, increased hospital bed availability for sicker patients, minimization of separation from parents and reduction of hospital-acquired infections.

❑❑ What are the most important defense mechanisms of the lung against environmental and infectious agents?

Mucociliary transport and the cough reflex.

❑❑ How is the cough reflex impaired after surgery?

It is inhibited by pain and the use of narcotic analgesia. In addition, respiratory muscle dysfunction reduces the expulsive force and the effectiveness of the cough.

❑❑ How long after general anesthesia is the mucociliary clearance reduced?

For 2 to 6 days. This is the result of ciliary damage from dry anesthetic gases, increased mucus viscosity and reduced clearance from areas of atelectasis.

❏❏ **When should intermittent positive pressure breathing (IPPB) be used?**

IPPB is best reserved for those patients where active lung inflation is not possible even with patient cooperation (e.g., muscular dystrophy, kyphoscoliosis).

❏❏ **What is the net effect of the shift from diaphragmatic to intercostal breathing?**

Ventilation is redistributed and less inspiratory gas is delivered to the lower lobes, decreased FRC and decreased closing capacity. The net result is atelectasis.

❏❏ **What are the clinical characteristics of malignant hyperthermia?**

Muscular rigidity, fever, tachycardia, respiratory and metabolic acidosis, severe hypermetabolism, arrhythmias and eventual hypotension and cardiovascular collapse.

❏❏ **What is the incidence of elevated left hemidiaphragm when an internal mammary artery graft is used?**

39%.

❏❏ **How long do changes in respiratory function last following thoracotomy?**

Up to 3 weeks.

❏❏ **What is the mechanism of action of nondepolarizing neuromuscular blocking agents?**

They combine with nicotinic cholinergic postjunctional receptors. However, they do not activate the receptor or directly block the channel.

❏❏ **Why is there such widespread popularity for the use of propofol in ambulatory anesthesia?**

Its effects dissipate rapidly, it has a lower incidence of postoperative nausea and vomiting, a high degree of patient satisfaction and minimal side effects.

❏❏ **How does propofol affect the cardiovascular system?**

It causes cardiovascular depression by direct myocardial effects and vasodilatation.

❏❏ **What patients should receive prophylactic dantrolene?**

Those with a prior history of malignant hyperthermia and those proven to be at risk (determined by muscle biopsy).

❏❏ **T/F: Propofol is contraindicated in patients with an egg allergy.**

True.

❏❏ **What effect does thoracotomy have on respiratory system compliance?**

Compliance may decrease by as much as 75%, which markedly increases the work of breathing.

❏❏ **What are the effects of sternotomy compared to lateral thoracotomy on postoperative pulmonary function?**

Less postoperative pain and discomfort and more rapid return of pulmonary function.

❏❏ **T/F: Carboxyhemoglobin produces an artificially elevated reading of oxygen saturation.**

True.

❏❏ **What anatomic changes occur after pneumonectomy?**

The mediastinum shifts, the hemi-diaphragm elevates, the rib interspaces become smaller on the operated side, the remaining lung distends to fill the space and the remaining space fills with connective tissue.

❏❏ **What are the benefits of intraoperative analgesic compounds?**

They improve hemodynamic stability, decrease the anesthetic requirement, provide for a more rapid emergence from anesthesia and decrease postoperative pain and discomfort.

❏❏ **What are the advantages of epidural anesthesia?**

Earlier mobilization and return of bowel function, shorter hospital stay, decreased sedation and decreased stress response to surgery.

❏❏ **What drug is used to reverse the effects of narcotics?**

Naloxone.

❏❏ **What is the mechanism of action of local anesthetics?**

They temporarily block nerve conduction by binding to neuronal sodium channels.

❏❏ **What are the risk factors for postoperative pulmonary complications?**

The anatomic site for surgery, general debility of the patient, presence of chronic obstructive lung disease, obesity (>120 kg.), cigarette smoking and preoperative hypercapnia.

❏❏ **What are the mechanisms of post extubation airway closure?**

Laryngeal edema, laryngospasm and failure of vocal cord abduction.

❏❏ **What are the effects of benzodiazepines?**

Anxiolysis, sedation and anterograde amnesia.

❏❏ **What is the mechanism of halothane-induced cardiac arrythmias?**

Halothane sensitizes the heart to endogenous and exogenous catecholamines.

❏❏ **What are the undesirable effects of midazolam in elderly or debilitated patients?**

Substantial sedation, respiratory depression and hypoxemia.

❏❏ **What is the benzodiazepine-specific antagonist?**

Flumazenil (Romazicon).

❏❏ **T/F: Pulse oximetry measures arterial oxygen tension (PaO_2).**

False.

❏❏ **How does diazepam differ from midazolam?**

Diazepam is about one-fifth as potent, longer-acting, (elimination half-life of 20 to 40 hours) and less expensive.

❑❑ **What should be told to a mother who is concerned about the risk of intraoperative death in her otherwise healthy 15 year old son having ambulatory orthopedic surgery?**

The overall mortality associated with anesthesia and surgery is very low and when it does occur, it is usually unavoidable and due to progression of the presenting condition.

❑❑ **T/F: The extrapyramidal side effects of droperidol are nonexistent at low doses (0.625 to 1.25 mg).**

False.

❑❑ **What are the neurologic effects of ketamine?**

It produces a state of dissociation characterized by intense analgesia, a blank stare, nystagmus, amnesia, normal body tone, mild sedation and postemergence delirium.

❑❑ **How does flumazenil affect the amnestic properties of medazolam?**

Intraoperative amnesia is maintained while postoperative amnesia is terminated after flumazenil is given.

❑❑ **Which local anesthetic produces toxicity at the lowest dose?**

Tetracaine.

❑❑ **What is the onset of action of intravenous fentanyl?**

Within 2 minutes.

❑❑ **What is the standard of care in intraoperative blood pressure monitoring?**

Intermittent, noninvasive measurement with an oscillometric blood pressure cuff.

❑❑ **What is the duration of the analgesic properties of fentanyl?**

Approximately 45 minutes.

❑❑ **What are the side effects of opioid analgesics?**

Respiratory depression, pruritis, bradycardia, spasm of skeletal and smooth muscle, nausea and vomiting, constipation, ileus, urinary retention, physical dependence, orthostatic hypotension and histamine release.

❑❑ **Why does halothane have a relatively high uptake by fat and cause relatively slow emergence?**

It has a high blood-gas and blood-tissue solubility.

❑❑ **T/F: Succinylcholine is a depolarizing muscle relaxant.**

True.

❑❑ **How would you determine a loading dose for a drug to reach an effective plasma concentration quickly?**

The loading dose is equal to the product of the desired plasma concentration and the volume of distribution.

❏❏ **What local anesthetic is the greatest offender of transient radicular irritation (TRI)?**

Lidocaine.

❏❏ **When is intraoperative arterial blood pressure measure indicated?**

When tight control is required, e.g., patients with significant hypertension, serious cardiac disease, significant acute blood loss and those with left ventricular dysfunction who are undergoing extended surgical procedures with significant fluid shifts and potential blood loss.

❏❏ **What receptor does succinylcholine target?**

The postjunctional nicotinic cholinergic receptor.

❏❏ **How is the action of succinylcholine terminated?**

By hydrolysis of plasma pseudocholinesterase.

❏❏ **What is the mechanism of action of nonsteroidal anti-inflammatory agents (NSAIDs)?**

They act primarily through peripheral inhibition of prostaglandin synthesis. The cyclooxygenase enzyme is inhibited, reducing the conversion of arachidonic acid to cyclic endoperoxide. Decreased production of arachidonic metabolites limits inflammation and perceived pain while avoiding opioid chemoreceptor stimulation and its attendant side effects.

❏❏ **What is the presumed mechanism of action of the antiemetic effect of ephedrine in the postoperative period?**

It increases sympathetic tone, thus, minimizing postoperative nausea and vomiting secondary to a high degree of vagal tone.

❏❏ **What are the effects of viral URI's on lung function in the pediatric population?**

Decreased FVC, FEV1, PEFR and MMEF.

❏❏ **What is the major determinant of a patient's risk for perioperative complications?**

The specific surgical procedure to be performed.

❏❏ **What are the advantages of intravenous regional anesthesia?**

It is easily performed and rapidly resolves with tourniquet release.

❏❏ **What advantages do infusion techniques offer over bolus techniques?**

A steady state is more easily achieved, peaks and valleys of anesthetic levels are minimized and the total amount of drug required to produce anesthesia is reduced.

❏❏ **What peripheral nerve of the brachial plexus can be potentially spared after performing an interscalene block?**

The ulnar nerve.

❏❏ **What are the discharge criteria following ambulatory surgery?**

Stable vital signs, ability to ambulate, intact protective airway reflexes, adequate hydration with the ability to hold down oral intake and adequate pain control.

❏❏ **Which potent inhalation anesthetic is associated with seizure activity?**

Enflurane.

❏❏ **How is remifentanil metabolized?**

By non-specific blood and tissue esterases, resulting in an ultra-short terminal half-life of 10 minutes.

❏❏ **What are the physiologic parameters measured by the Apache II score?**

Temperature, respiratory rate, heart rate, arterial pH, serum levels of potassium, sodium and creatinine, hematocrit, oxygenation, white blood cell count and Glascow Coma Scale.

❏❏ **What is the origin of the brachial plexus?**

The anterior primary divisions of C5 through T1.

❏❏ **What peripheral nerve of the brachial plexus is most commonly spared in an axillary block?**

The musculocutaneous nerve.

❏❏ **The interscalene block is performed at what level of the brachial plexus?**

The roots.

❏❏ **How do you test motor block of the median nerve?**

Opposition of the thumb (opponens pollicus).

❏❏ **How would you test motor block of the musculocutaneous nerve?**

Flexion at the elbow (biceps brachialis and corachobrachialis).

❏❏ **The spinal cord typically ends at what level?**

L1 or L2.

❏❏ **What complications are associated with spinal anesthesia?**

Hypotension, bradycardia, postspinal headache, nausea, urinary retention, backache, neurologic sequelae and hypoventilation.

❏❏ **Inherited abnormalities of what enzyme contributes to respiratory insufficiency with succinylcholine administration?**

Serum cholinesterase.

❏❏ **What are the disadvantages of continuous spinal anesthesia?**

Additional time is required to place the catheter, spinal headache and potential for catheter breakage, infection, nerve trauma and hemorrhage.

❏❏ **How is atracurium metabolized?**

It undergoes spontaneous degradation (Hoffman) at body pH and temperature and by ester hydrolysis.

❏❏ **What are the essential components of conscious sedation?**

Amnesia, sedation and analgesia.

☐☐ **What pharmacologic factors create the ideal drug for intravenous sedation?**

Water solubility, non-irritating, rapid onset, short duration of action, readily titratable effect, ease of administration, absence of cardiovascular or respiratory depressant effects, no hypersensitivity reaction, non-organ-dependent elimination, absence of toxicity, pharmacokinetics independent of altered physiology, rapid recovery and a favorable cost-benefit ratio.

☐☐ **What equation allows rapid calculation of approximate endotracheal tube size in the pediatric patient?**

(Age / 4) + 4 = internal diameter of the ETT.

☐☐ **What pharmacokinetic property of nitrous oxide makes induction and emergence with this agent rapid?**

It has a low blood gas solubility.

☐☐ **Why is pain experienced with intravenous administration of thiopental?**

Because of its alkaline pH (between 10 and 11).

☐☐ **What are the side effects of etomidate?**

Myoclonus, pain on injection, nausea and vomiting and adrenal suppression.

☐☐ **What are the disadvantages of nitrous oxide?**

It readily diffuses into gas-containing spaces in the body, can contribute to perioperative nausea and vomiting and has a low potency when used alone.

☐☐ **What monitoring does the ASA recommend for anesthetic care?**

Oxygenation, ventilation, circulation and temperature must be continually evaluated.

CRITICAL CARE, SHOCK, FLUIDS AND ELECTROLYTE PEARLS

Nature heals, under the auspices of the medical profession.
Haven Emerson

❑❑ T/F: Colloid solutions are preferred for resuscitation.

False.

❑❑ How is stroke volume (SV) determined?

Ejection fraction (EF) x heart rate (HR).

❑❑ What parameter measured by pulmonary artery (PA) catheters correlates with response to a fluid challenge?

Right ventricular end-diastolic volume (RVEDV) less than 140 correlates in a positive fashion with increased cardiac output (CO) upon fluid challenge.

❑❑ T/F: Blood products should be given as the initial resuscitation fluid for patients with presumed large blood loss.

False.

❑❑ What parameters indicate successful resuscitation?

Return of normal vital signs and signs of end-organ perfusion (i.e., urine output and clear mentation).

❑❑ What are the indications for central venous cannulation?

As a conduit for PA catheters, lack of peripheral access, CVP monitoring and infusion of vasoactive medications or medications requiring high flow veins, including TPN.

❑❑ What is the preferred site for central venous catheterization?

Controversial. All three major sites (femoral, internal jugular and subclavian) have advantages and disadvantages.

❑❑ What are the most common immediate complications of central venous catheterization?

Pneumothorax, hemothorax, arrhythmias, arterial puncture, air embolus and malposition.

❑❑ What are the common delayed complications from central venous catheterization?

Infection, thrombus formation, erosion through the superior vena cava (SVC) or atrium and delayed pneumothorax.

❑❑ What catheter tip culture result is suggestive of catheter sepsis?

Greater than 15 colonies of the same organism.

❑❑ **A diagnosis of nosocomial pneumonia is based primarily on what criteria?**

The development of a new infiltrate, new onset of purulent sputum and isolation of a pathogen from blood culture, transtracheal aspirate or bronchial brushing or biopsy.

❑❑ **Aminoslycosides are effective against which bacteria?**

Aerobic gram negative bacilli (including Pseudomonas aeruginosa), enterococci, staphlococci and streptococci.

❑❑ **What risks are associated with the use of aminoglycosides?**

Prolonged neuromuscular blockade, ototoxicity and nephrotoxicity.

❑❑ **Vancomycin is effective against which bacteria?**

Gram-positive cocci, including methicillin-resistant Staphyloccocus aureus (MRSA), Staphylococcus epidermidis, enterococcus, diptheroids and Clostridium difficile.

❑❑ **T/F: Treatment for Clostridium difficile may include oral vancomycin.**

True.

❑❑ **What is Red Man's Syndrome?**

Flushing of the face and neck, pruritis and hypotension associated with rapid infusion of vancomycin and subsequent release of histamine.

❑❑ **What more recent problem has arisen with the use of vancomycin?**

Development of vancomycin resistant enterococci (VRE).

❑❑ **What agents are used to treat VRE?**

Chloramphenicol, novobiocin, synercid, teichoplanin, quinolones and doxycycline.

❑❑ **What factors determine cardiac output (CO)?**

Preload, afterload, contractility and heart rate.

❑❑ **What do alpha-2 and Dopamine-2 receptors have in common?**

They are presynaptic and function in a negative feedback loop such that their activation inhibits subsequent release of neurotransmitters.

❑❑ **T/F: Beta-blockers affect the serum potassium concentration.**

True. They inhibit uptake of potassium by skeletal muscle.

❑❑ **What is the treatment for autonomic hyperreflexia?**

Eliminate the predisposing factor(s) and administration of antihypertensives ganglionic blockers.

❑❑ **What is the most common metabolic acid/base derangement seen in SICU patients?**

Metabolic alkalosis.

❑❑ **What is the basal production of lactic acid?**

Approximately 1,440 mEq/day.

❑❑ **How is the fractional excretion of sodium (FeNa) calculated?**

FeNa = [(Una / Pna) / (Ucr / Pcr)] X 100%.

❑❑ **What is the definition of preload?**

End-diastolic sarcoma length.

❑❑ **What is the most reliable test for differentiation of acute oliguric renal failure from prerenal azotemia?**

The FeNa (greater than 2% in acute renal failure and less than 1% in prerenal azotemia).

❑❑ **Diabetes insipidus (DI) infers what tonicity of urine and plasma?**

Dilute urine and a hypertonic plasma osmolality.

❑❑ **What is the major cause of extrarenal potassium depletion?**

Diarrhea.

❑❑ **What are the clinical manifestations of hypokalemia?**

Muscle weakness, mental status changes, impaired intestinal peristalsis and predisposition to digitalis toxicity.

❑❑ **Deficiency of phosphorous may affect oxygen transfer from erythrocytes as a result of its contribution to what compound?**

2,3-diphosphoglycerate (2,3-DPG).

❑❑ **T/F: The pulmonary capillary wedge pressure (PCWP) is a reflection of left atrial pressure.**

True.

❑❑ **What is the role of chromium in human metabolism?**

It promotes the effects of insulin on peripheral tissues.

❑❑ **What are ECG changes frequently associated with hyperkalemia?**

A widened QRS and PR interval, peaked T waves, flattened P waves, deep S waves, ventricular tachycardia or fibrillation and asystole.

❑❑ **Compensation for persistent hypoventilation occurs by what mechanism?**

Resorption of sodium bicarbonate by the kidney.

❑❑ **How do inotropic agents increase myocardial contractility?**

By increasing intracellular calcium concentration and availability.

❑❑ **In the surgical patient, metabolic acidosis is frequently caused by circulatory failure and accumulation of lactic acid. What is the appropriate treatment for this?**

Assuming an adequate cardiac output, volume resuscitation with fluid or blood restores circulation and hepatic clearance of lactate.

❏❏ **What ECG abnormalities are associated with hypercalcemia?**

A shortened Q-T interval, bradycardia and heart block.

❏❏ **At normal body temperature, what is the average daily insensible water loss?**

600 to 900 ml/day or 8 to 12 ml/kg/day.

❏❏ **What are the consequences of exceedingly rapid sodium replacement in patients with hyponatremia?**

Central pontine myelinolysis (i.e., quadriplegia, dysarthria and dysphasia).

❏❏ **What are the common causes of hyperosmolar hyponatremia?**

Hyperglycemia, mannitol and radiologic contrast.

❏❏ **Patients with asymptomatic hyponatremia are best treated in what manner?**

Free water restriction.

❏❏ **What level of urine sodium may distinguish extrarenal from renal sodium loss, contributing to hyponatremia?**

Less than 20 mEq/l.

❏❏ **What are the most common pathogens associated with catheter-related sepsis?**

Staphylococcus aureus and epidermidis, candida, klebsiella, enterobacter, pseudomonas and enterococci.

❏❏ **What is the arterial-venous oxygen difference a measure of?**

The extent to which blood flow matches the metabolic demand for oxygen.

❏❏ **What are the indications for invasive arterial monitoring?**

Need for constant pressure monitoring due to a dynamic clinical picture, vasoactive medications and need for frequent arterial blood gas monitoring.

❏❏ **What are the preferred and acceptable alternative sites for arterial lines?**

The radial artery is preferred due to a high degree of collateral flow to the hand. Femoral, dorsalis pedis and axillary arteries are acceptable.

❏❏ **T/F: Non invasive arterial pressure measurements are more accurate than direct arterial measurements.**

False.

❏❏ **What patient populations are most likely to be helped by the use of a PA catheter?**

Patients with myocardial infarction and shock and those with shock refractory to volume loading, perioperative management of patients undergoing cardiac or vascular surgery and multiple trauma patients.

❏❏ **What complications are associated with the use of PA catheters?**

All possible complications inherent in any central venous access, as well as pulmonary artery rupture, a higher incidence of arrhythmias and knotting of the catheter.

❑❑ **What is the normal mixed venous blood oxygen saturation (MVO_2)?**

Approximately 75%.

❑❑ **How is arterial oxygen content (CaO_2) calculated?**

CaO_2 = (Hgb x 1.39) x SaO_2 + (PaO_2 x 0.0031).

❑❑ **What are the typical PA catheter measurements in early septic shock?**

High CO, low systemic vascular resistance (SVR) and high PCWP. In later stages, the CO will drop and SVR may rise.

❑❑ **What is the treatment for patients in septic shock?**

Volume infusion. Once euvolemia is achieved, inotropic support should be considered. However, the ultimate treatment is locating and removing the source of sepsis.

❑❑ **How is cardiogenic shock managed?**

Euvolemia first, then inotropic support.

❑❑ **What are typical PA catheter measurements in neurogenic shock?**

High or low CO, low SVR and low PCWP.

❑❑ **How is neurogenic shock managed?**

Volume infusion followed by pressors, if needed.

❑❑ **What is the most important factor in control of ventilation under normal conditions?**

$PaCO_2$.

❑❑ **What are the characteristics of dopamine?**

It is a dopaminergic and beta-1 agonist at low doses and an alpha-agonist at higher doses.

❑❑ **What is the major difference between dopamine and dobutamine?**

Dobutamine lacks alpha-1 effects.

❑❑ **What are the major differences between epinephrine and norepinephrine?**

Epinephrine has mostly beta effects, norepinephrine has mostly alpha.

❑❑ **How is oxygen delivery (DO_2) calculated?**

DO_2 = CI x CaO_2 x 10.

❑❑ **What is transpulmonary pressure?**

The pressure gradient across the lung measured as the pressure difference between the airway opening and the pleural surface.

❏❏ **Which pulmonary function test is least dependent on patient effort?**

Forced expiratory flow 25 to 75% (FEV_{25-75}).

❏❏ **What is the primary form of carbon dioxide transport in the circulation?**

Carbon dioxide hydrolyzed by carbonic anhydrase to carbonic acid.

❏❏ **What are the most common causes of the syndrome of inappropriate antidiuretic hormone (SIADH)?**

Malignancies, pulmonary disease, CNS disorders and drugs.

❏❏ **What is the treatment for patients with diabetes insipidus (DI)?**

Vasopressin intravenously or DDAVP intranasally. Chronic therapy with chloropropramide (stimulates ADH release) and thiazide diuretics has been used successfully.

❏❏ **How fast should hyponatremia be corrected?**

No faster than 0.5 to 1.0 mEq/l/hour.

❏❏ **How is urine osmolality calculated?**

Urine osmolality = 2 x (urinary sodium + urinary potassium) + (urine urea nitrogen / 2.8).

❏❏ **What are the significant clinical manifestations of hyperkalemia?**

Neuromuscular weakness that may progress to flaccid paralysis and hypoventilation.

❏❏ **What ECG changes are associated with hypokalemia?**

A decreased T wave amplitude, prominent U waves, QRS prolongation, P wave changes, cardiac arrhythmias and AV block.

❏❏ **How is body potassium distributed?**

90% is intracellular (mainly in muscle), 2% is extracellular and the remainder is in bone.

❏❏ **How is oxygen consumption (VO_2) calculated?**

VO_2 = CI x C(a - v)O_2 x 10.

❏❏ **How does dopamine promote diuresis?**

Low-dose dopamine (2 to 4 mcg/kg/min) binds to dopaminergic receptors and increases renal blood flow. It also directly inhibits sodium resorption in the proximal tubule. Even at those low doses, beta-adrenergic activation increases cardiac contractility, which also increases renal blood flow.

❏❏ **What are the most common causes of hypernatremia?**

DI, insensible losses, osmotic diuresis and hypertonic fluid administration.

❏❏ **How does acute metabolic alkalosis affect serum potassium?**

Plasma potassium falls by 0.3 mEq/l for every 0.1 unit rise in pH.

❏❏ **What therapy is available for patients with severe hyperkalemia?**

Calcium, sodium bicarbonate, beta-adrenergic agonists, cation exchange resins, loop diuretics, insulin and glucose and dialysis (definitive treatment).

❏❏ **What factors can potentially contribute to the difficulty in weaning critically ill patients from mechanical ventilation?**

Lack of central ventilatory drive due to encephalopathy, primary septic myopathy, muscle fatigue or weakness and neuropathy of critical illness.

❏❏ **Respiratory failure is worsened in spinal injuries at or above which nerve root?**

C2.

❏❏ **What infectious syndromes can lead to ventilatory insufficiency?**

Botulism, tetanus, campylobacter, polio, diphtheria and Guillain Barré Syndrome.

❏❏ **What is considered a normal Allen test?**

Palmar blush within 7 seconds of ulnar artery release.

❏❏ **Adequacy of alveolar ventilation is reflected by which component of arterial blood gas analysis?**

$PaCO_2$.

❏❏ **$PaCO_2$ is mathematically related to alveolar ventilation in what manner?**

Inverse proportion.

❏❏ **What factors interfere with the bellows function of the chest?**

Abdominal binding, massive obesity, trauma with flail chest, massive effusion and ascites, pneumothorax, thoracic burn with eschar, neuromuscular blockade and strapping of ribs.

❏❏ **What is the principal mechanism of increased $PaCO_2$ with increased FIO_2?**

Worsening V/Q mismatch and the Haldane effect.

❏❏ **How does malnutrition contribute to respiratory failure?**

Increase in the oxygen cost of breathing and respiratory muscle weakness.

❏❏ **How does positive end-expiratory pressure (PEEP) decrease cardiac output?**

It decreases preload.

❏❏ **In which lung zone should a pulmonary artery catheter tip be located?**

Zone III.

❏❏ **Which lobes of the lung can develop atelectasis from intubation of the right mainstem bronchus?**

The right upper lobe, left upper lobe and left lower lobe.

❏❏ **What are the determinants of $PaCO_2$?**

Carbon dioxide production and alveolar ventilation.

❏❏ **What are the primary determinants of the oxygen content of arterial blood?**

The product of hemoglobin concentration and the percent hemoglobin oxygen saturation of arterial blood.

❏❏ **How long does it take to demonstrate the earliest manifestations of oxygen toxicity while breathing 100% oxygen?**

1 to 2 hours.

❏❏ **What are the components of tidal volume?**

Alveolar volume and dead space volume.

❏❏ **What factor limits the ability to reliably deliver an FIO_2 > 35% via a Venturi mask?**

Inability to deliver a sufficient flow rate of oxygen.

❏❏ **What is the maximum acceptable endotracheal tube cuff pressure?**

Approximately 26 cm H_2O at end-expiration.

❏❏ **What are the indications for mechanical ventilatory support?**

Respiratory rate greater than 35, $PaCO_2$ greater than 60 mm Hg, (A-a) O_2 greater than 350 mm Hg and VD/VT greater than 0.6.

❏❏ **What is the potential harm of excess endotracheal tube cuff pressure?**

It can induce ischemia and necrosis of the underlying tissue.

❏❏ **What are the mechanisms of obstructive shock?**

Impedance to filling (e.g., tamponade and restrictive cardiomyopathies) and impedance to outflow (e.g., valvular stenoses).

❏❏ **What is the classic hemodynamic finding of cardiac tamponade?**

Equalization of the diastolic pressures of the heart chambers.

❏❏ **Why does removal of very little pericardial fluid in tamponade greatly improve the clinical picture?**

Tamponade occurs at the right side of the pericardial compliance curve where small changes in volume cause large changes in pressure.

❏❏ **What causes electrical alternans on the ECG of a patient with cardiac tamponade?**

Cyclic motion of the heart in the fluid filled pericardial sac.

❏❏ **What clinical findings are likely to be seen in a patient with cardiac tamponade?**

Beck's triad (muffled heart tones, distended neck veins and hypotension).

❏❏ **What is the etiology pulsus paradoxus?**

A greater than normal decrease in systolic arterial pressure with inspiration.

❏❏ **What is the differential diagnosis for pulsus paradoxus?**

Cardiac tamponade, status asthmaticus, severe chronic obstructive lung disease, pulmonary embolus, constrictive pericarditis and tension pneumothorax.

❏❏ **What clinical finding distinguishes cardiac tamponade from constrictive pericarditis?**

Kussmaul's sign (increase in venous pressure during inspiration) is not seen in tamponade.

❏❏ **What is the most common clinical finding in cardiac tamponade?**

Tachypnea (80%), followed by pulsus paradoxus (77%) and tachycardia (77%).

❏❏ **What is the differential diagnosis for a patient with recurrent pulmonary or systemic embolization and acute cardiogenic shock?**

End-stage dilated cardiomyopathy or atrial myxoma.

❏❏ **Which parameter, obtained on routine vital signs, usually indicates a hypodynamic state?**

A narrowed pulse pressure.

❏❏ **What are the underlying pathogenetic mechanisms of cardiogenic shock?**

Loss of contractile muscle, valvular failure, dysrhythmias and myocardial rupture.

❏❏ **What is the classic clinical sign of systolic ventricular dysfunction?**

An S3 gallop.

❏❏ **Can preload and PCWP be used as synonyms?**

No. PCWP is determined by juxtaventricular pressures, ventricular compliance and left ventricular end-diastolic volume (LVEDV). LVEDV and preload are synonyms.

❏❏ **T/F: Septal rupture occurs more commonly in anterior infarcts than in inferior infarcts.**

False. The incidence is approximately the same.

❏❏ **Why does the posteromedial papillary muscle ruptures most often?**

It is perfused from only one of the coronary arteries, whereas the anterolateral papillary muscle is perfused from the left and right coronary circulation.

❏❏ **What major conditions are associated with distributive shock?**

Sepsis, anaphylaxis, neurogenic shock and adrenal insufficiency.

❏❏ **What are the key endogenous molecular mediators of septic shock?**

Cytokines (mainly TNF-alpha, IL-1, IL-6 and IFN-gamma), prostaglandins, complement, platelet-activating factor and nitric oxide.

❏❏ **What is the pathogenesis of anaphylactic shock?**

Anaphylactic shock is an extreme manifestation of an immediate hypersensitivity reaction. It occurs through the interaction of an inciting antigen with mast cells and basophil-bound IgE. These effector cells then release numerous pre-stored and newly synthesized mediators that produce the clinical findings.

❏❏ **What are the effects of septic shock on cardiac function?**

There is transient dilatation of one or both ventricles, reduced contractility and a low ejection fraction. These changes typically last several days and normalize after 7 to 10 days.

❏❏ **What are the typical clinical findings that distinguish distributive shock from other types of shock?**

Warm, well-perfused skin, a wide pulse pressure and a reduced diastolic blood pressure.

❏❏ **What degree of blood loss is required to induce hypotension?**

20 to 25% of the blood volume.

❏❏ **What are the typical values of mixed venous oxygen saturation (MVO_2) in septic shock?**

It is often elevated above normal secondary to inadequate oxygen extraction by tissues.

❏❏ **T/F: The finding of a hyperdynamic hemodynamic profile can confirm or exclude a septic etiology of shock.**

False.

❏❏ **What are the initial priorities during shock resuscitation?**

Stabilization and cause-specific correction of systemic and regional circulatory failure.

❏❏ **What are the physiological goals of shock resuscitation?**

Correction of oxygen debt, anaerobic metabolism and tissue acidosis.

❏❏ **What is the importance of the splanchnic area during shock and the post-shock phase?**

The splanchnic tissues are preferentially underperfused relative to their metabolic demands during shock. Left uncorrected, it is associated with increased morbidity and mortality.

❏❏ **What is the initial blood pressure goal in shock resuscitation?**

Mean arterial pressure (MAP) of at least 60 to 70 mm Hg.

❏❏ **What is the significance of blood lactate determination in shock patients?**

Mortality is directly related to the degree of lactic acidosis.

❏❏ **How should the PCWP be used to guide fluid resuscitation in shock?**

Serial PCWP determinations following fluid challenges may indicate the limit of the cardiovascular system to accept further volume expansion without adverse effects.

❏❏ **T/F: A normal cardiac output exclude cardiac dysfunction.**

False.

❏❏ **What is the optimal hematocrit in shock patients?**

Approximately 30%.

❏❏ **What is the role of catecholamines in the resuscitation of shock?**

Inotropic and/or vasopressor support once effective intravascular volume has been restored.

❏❏ **What are the major drawbacks of catecholamine use in shock?**

Catecholamines can increase myocardial and systemic oxygen demands, induce arrhythmias and cause excessive vasoconstriction, resulting in ischemia.

❏❏ **T/F: Normalization of vital signs, such as blood pressure and heart rate indicate completed resuscitation of shock.**

False. Systemic vital signs do not reliably reflect the physiologic end-points of shock resuscitation.

❏❏ **What is the most common proximate cause of death in shock patients?**

Multiple organ failure (MOF).

❏❏ **What are the most common presenting findings in adult/acute respiratory distress syndrome (ARDS)?**

Tachypnea and hypoxemia.

❏❏ **What cellular mediators are involved in the development of ARDS?**

Tumor necrosis factor (TNF), IL-1 and arachidonic acid.

❏❏ **What are the NIH criteria for the diagnosis of ARDS?**

A PaO_2/FIO_2 ratio less than 200, bilateral infiltrates and a wedge pressure less than 18.

❏❏ **What is the cause of hypoxemia in ARDS?**

An increase in alveolar fluid causing reduced diffusion of oxygen into capillaries, thus, increasing the shunt.

❏❏ **What is the mortality rate for patients with ARDS?**

40 to 60%.

❏❏ **What are the most common risk factors associated with ARDS?**

Sepsis, trauma, aspiration, multiple transfusions, shock and pulmonary contusions.

❏❏ **Why is the PCWP an important feature in the diagnosis of ARDS?**

The presence of a significantly elevated wedge pressure infers that the pulmonary edema may be hydrostatic and, therefore, due to LV dysfunction rather than alveolar or pulmonary dysfunction and ARDS (e.g., noncardiogenic pulmonary edema).

❏❏ **What is the characteristic histologic alveolar change in patients with ARDS?**

Type 1 alveolar surface cells, which are sensitive to injury, are destroyed and replaced with Type 2 alveolar cells and cellular debris.

❏❏ **What is the distribution of pulmonary edema in ARDS?**

Routine chest x-rays show a diffuse distribution. However, CT scan studies reveal an increased involvement in the dependent portions of the lung fields.

❏❏ **What are the x-ray findings in ARDS?**

Bilateral, diffuse ground glass-like infiltrates that do not follow anatomical boundaries.

❏❏ **What complications are associated with ARDS?**

Barotrauma, pulmonary infection, pulmonary hypertension and MOF.

❏❏ **What is the advantage of pressure-controlled ventilation in ARDS?**

It allows for higher mean airway pressures and better oxygenation with relatively lower peak airway pressures.

❏❏ **What are the phases of ARDS?**

Acute or exudative (up to 6 days), proliferative (4 to 10 days) and chronic or fibrotic (after 7 days).

❏❏ **What is the role of PEEP in ARDS?**

Maintenance of alveolar inflation and functional residual capacity (FRC).

❏❏ **What is compliance and how is it calculated?**

Compliance is the measure of the elasticity of the lungs. It is calculated by measuring the change in volume divided by the change in pressure.

❏❏ **What are the negative effects of PEEP on cardiovascular function?**

PEEP may reduce the cardiac output by reducing venous return, increasing pulmonary vascular resistance and shifting the intraventricular septum to the left, thus, reducing the LVEDV.

❏❏ **What is the closing capacity of the lungs?**

The lung volume at which small airways close.

❏❏ **What is the predominant stimulus for activation of hypoxic pulmonary vasoconstriction?**

Decreased alveolar oxygen tension.

❏❏ **What are the most common initial rhythms in adults with cardiac arrest?**

Ventricular fibrillation (VF) and ventricular tachycordia (VT).

❏❏ **For VF or unstable VT, what is the most important intervention to optimize chances for successful resuscitation?**

Defibrillation.

❏❏ **What is the primary indication for atropine?**

Symptomatic bradycardia.

❏❏ **A 28 year old male presents with hemodynamically stable paroxysmal supraventricular tachycardia (PSVT) at a rate of 170. What is the drug of choice?**

Vagal maneuvers are tried first. If unsuccessful, adenosine is the drug of choice.

❏❏ **What side effects are associated with adenosine?**

Transient ischemic-type chest pain, recurrence of supraventricular tachycardia and transient asystole.

❐❐ **What is the primary goal in treatment of rapid atrial fibrillation?**

To slow the ventricular response rate. In unstable patients, electrical conversion is the treatment of choice. In stable patients, beta-blockers and calcium channel blockers will slow AV conduction.

❐❐ **What is the treatment of choice for rapid atrial fibrillation in a patient with Wolff-Parkinson-White syndrome?**

Cardioversion if the patient is unstable, otherwise procainamide (20 to 30 mg/min up to 17 mg/kg). The infusion should be stopped if further widening of the QRS or hypotension occurs.

❐❐ **Calcium use is de-emphasized but is still indicated for which situations?**

Hyperkalemia, hypocalcemia and calcium channel blocker toxicity.

❐❐ **Why is bretylium a second line pharmacologic treatment for ventricular ectopy?**

Bretylium is associated with adverse hemodynamic effects.

❐❐ **A patient's temperature is 30° Celsius. During cardiac arrest defibrillation was unsuccessful. What treatment is recommend?**

Active warming should precede further defibrillation attempts and medication administration.

❐❐ **When should open chest massage be considered?**

Early in the treatment of penetrating chest trauma, in situations in which closed chest massage is ineffective or in which aortic cross-clamping may be beneficial.

❐❐ **What drugs may be given via the endotracheal tube?**

Lidocaine, atropine, naloxone and epinephrine.

❐❐ **What determines the relationship between changes in airway pressure and lung volume during positive-pressure ventilation?**

Lung and chest wall compliance.

❐❐ **T/F: Pleural pressure is equal throughout the thorax.**

False. There are hydrostatic pressure gradients from the dependent to non-dependent regions and surface-specific differences.

❐❐ **T/F: Acute lung injury of the entire lung causes lung compliance to decrease similarly in each region of the lung.**

False. Marked regional differences in the degree of lung consolidation and compliance characterize all forms of acute lung injury.

❐❐ **Under normal conditions at rest, what percentage of the cardiac output goes to the respiratory muscles?**

Less than 3%.

❐❐ **In patients with COPD, what percentage of the total cardiac output can be directed to the muscles of respiration?**

25 to 30%.

❏❏ **In patients with congestive heart failure (CHF), cardiovascular insufficiency and respiratory distress, the initiation of positive-pressure ventilation is often associated with what hemodynamic response?**

Improvement in overall cardiovascular status due to the combined effects of the reduced work of breathing and reduced LV afterload.

❏❏ **Weaning from mechanical ventilation is associated with what effect on myocardial oxygen demand?**

It increases it.

❏❏ **What signs and symptoms are associated with increased intracranial pressure (ICP)?**

Headache, nausea, emesis, papilledema, systemic hypertension, bradycardia, an irregular respiratory pattern and paralysis of upward gaze (setting sun sign).

❏❏ **What are the possible reasons for the development of postoperative hypokalemia?**

An intracellular shift secondary to high insulin or beta-agonist levels, hypothermia, hemodilution, hyperventilation, alkalosis, on-going diuresis and nasogastric suctioning

❏❏ **What is the relation between magnesium and potassium?**

Magnesium depletion promotes the loss of potassium in the urine, thus, its replacement helps to limit renal potassium wasting. Hypomagnesemia also inhibits sodium-potassium transport resulting in decreasing intracellular concentrations of potassium.

❏❏ **What complications are associated with hypothermia?**

Coagulopathy, confusion, disorientation, decreased immune response, platelet dysfunction, reduced cardiac function, decreased cardiac output, vasoconstriction and hypertension.

❏❏ **What measures can be instituted to treat hypothermia?**

Increasing the room temperature, using intravenous fluid and blood warmers, heating ventilator gases and using warming blankets.

❏❏ **As the patient re-warms, what problems can arise?**

Development of metabolic acidosis, shivering, hypotension and tachycardia.

❏❏ **An SICU trauma patient is noted to be oozing from multiple wound sites. What tests and accompanying results are consistent with disseminated intravascular coagulopathy (DIC)?**

A decreased platelet count, elevated prothrombin time (PT), elevated activated partial thromboplastin time (aPTT), decreased fibrinogen, elevated fibrin degradation products and presence of D-dimers.

❏❏ **What disorders are associated with auto-PEEP?**

Asthma, COPD and ARDS.

❏❏ **An intubated patient has been on 100% oxygen for 20 hours. What changes can be attributed to oxygen toxicity?**

Tracheobronchial irritation, decreased vital capacity, lung compliance, diffusion capacity and tracheal mucous viscosity, increased arteriovenous shunting and absorption atelectasis.

❏❏ **What is the pathophysiology of oxygen toxicity?**

Increased production of reactive oxygen metabolites. Production of free radicals exceeds the detoxification capacity of the superoxide dismutase system. The cytotoxic metabolites impair enzyme function and protein synthesis leading to decreased surfactant production, increased alveolar-capillary leakage, pulmonary edema and destruction of the capillary endothelium.

❏❏ **A patient has been ventilator dependent for 4 weeks and now appears to be making slow progress in weaning from the ventilator. What are the disadvantages of undergoing a tracheostomy?**

It requires the patient to undergo another surgical procedure and is associated with the risks of stoma granulation, tracheal erosion, tracheal stenosis and tracheo-innominate fistula.

❏❏ **What are the criteria for extubation?**

Tidal volume of at least 5 ml/kg, vital capacity of 15 ml/kg, negative inspiratory force less than -25 cm H2O, respiratory rate greater than 10 and less than 30, adequate oxygenation on an inspired oxygen concentration of 40% or less and ability to protect the airway.

❏❏ **Which patients are at risk for developing aspiration pneumonia?**

Patients undergoing emergency surgery, pregnant patients, obese patients, those with gastrointestinal obstruction, depressed level of consciousness and laryngeal incompetence.

❏❏ **What is the appropriate treatment following aspiration?**

Secure the airway, administer oxygen, suction any aspirate, consider bronchoscopy and lavage if large particulates are present, ventilatory support and bronchodilators as needed for bronchospasm.

❏❏ **A patient is admitted to the SICU after surgical debridement for necrotizing pancreatitis. Over the next several hours, his oxygenation deteriorates, with an oxygen saturation of 90% on 75% inspired oxygen and 10 of PEEP. What is the most likely diagnosis?**

ARDS.

❏❏ **What ventilatory steps could be taken to initially optimize the respiratory function in a patient with ARDS?**

Pressure control and inverse ratio ventilation, decrease the tidal volume and permissive hypercapnia.

❏❏ **What conditions or commonly used medications result in a decrease in serum theophylline concentration?**

Barbiturates, phenytoin, carbamazepine, rifampin, smoking and barbecued or smoked food consumption.

❏❏ **Given a 10% increase in Hgb, O_2 saturation and PaO_2, which is the most effective way to increase CaO_2?**

A 10% increase in Hgb.

❏❏ **What are the indicators of global oxygen transport insufficiency?**

A decrease in mixed oxygen saturation, increase in arterial-venous oxygen content difference and development of lactic acidosis.

❏❏ **What is heliox and when is it used?**

Helium has less density than oxygen and is thought to decrease the turbulence of flow past sites of obstruction. Heliox is a combination of helium and oxygen that is used when patients have an upper airway obstruction to decrease stridor, increase tidal volume and improve ventilation.

❏❏ **What are the clinical manifestations of the systemic inflammatory response syndrome (SIRS)?**

Fever or hypothermia, tachypnea, tachycardia, increased WBCs with a left shift and impaired organ perfusion.

❏❏ **What is the treatment for patients with SIRS?**

Fluid resuscitation, inotropic support, increased oxygen delivery and renal preservation techniques. Corticosteroids are NOT recommended.

❏❏ **Prophylaxis for stress ulcers includes what agents?**

Sucralfate, antacids and histamine receptor antagonists.

❏❏ **What are the risk factors for deep vein thrombosis (DVT)?**

Trauma or surgery to the pelvis or lower extremities, indwelling vascular catheters, prolonged immobility, a hypercoagulable state, lengthy anesthesia, RV failure, obesity, age over 50, cancer and the use of estrogen-containing compounds.

❏❏ **What preventive measures can be taken for patients at risk for developing a DVT?**

Early ambulation, elastic stockings that provide graded compression from ankle to thigh, low-dose heparin, intermittent pneumatic compression and prophylactic inferior vena cava filters.

❏❏ **What is the gold standard for diagnosis of pulmonary embolism (PE)?**

Pulmonary angiogram.

❏❏ **What patients are at high risk for complications during pulmonary angiogram?**

Those with recent myocardial infarction, severe pulmonary hypertension and arrhythmias. Safety can be improved with selective injections.

❏❏ **What are the indications for pulmonary angiography?**

Non-diagnostic, non-invasive venous studies, non-diagnostic V/Q scans, patients at high risk for anticoagulation and anticipated inferior vena cava filter placement, thrombolytic therapy or embolectomy.

❏❏ **What are the indications for inferior vena cava filter placement?**

A contraindication to anticoagulation, hemorrhage after anticoagulation, failure of anticoagulation to prevent recurrent PE and prophylaxis for extremely high-risk patients.

❏❏ **T/F: Total body water estimates should be decreased by 20 to 30% in obese patients.**

True.

❏❏ **Extracellular fluid comprises what percentage of total body water?**

30 to 33%.

☐☐ **T/F: Serum sodium is increased in the hyperglycemic patient.**

False. Hyperosmolar extracellular fluid shifts body water from the intracellular to the extracellular space. For each 100 mg/dl increase in glucose, sodium decreases 1.5 mEq/l.

☐☐ **Osmoreceptors in the hypothalamus control what two primary regulators of water balance?**

Thirst and ADH secretion.

☐☐ **A patient admitted with 1 week of persistent vomiting from gastric outlet obstruction is expected to have what acid-base disturbance?**

A hypokalemic, hypochloremic metabolic alkalosis.

☐☐ **What is the most common underlying disorder in respiratory acidosis?**

Alveolar hypoventilation.

☐☐ **How much sodium is in normal saline?**

154 mEq/l.

☐☐ **What is the daily fluid requirement for a 70 kg man?**

Approximately 2500 ml.

☐☐ **What are the clinical manifestations of hyponatremia?**

Weakness, fatigue, muscle cramps, confusion, anorexia, nausea, vomiting, headache, delirium, seizures and coma.

☐☐ **At what serum sodium level would one expect to see clinical signs and symptoms of acute hyponatremia?**

Approximately 125 mEq/l.

☐☐ **At what sodium level would one expect to see signs and symptoms of hypernatremia?**

Greater than 160 mEq/l.

☐☐ **What are the signs and symptoms of hypernatremia?**

Restlessness, irritability, ataxia, fever, spasms and seizure.

☐☐ **T/F: Elderly patients may have urine sodium levels that are inappropriately high in the face of decreased renal blood flow.**

True.

☐☐ **What is the urine sodium level and plasma osmolality in patients with SIADH?**

A urine sodium greater than 20 mEq/l and plasma osmolality less than 290 mOsm/l.

☐☐ **Hypocalcemia is associated with what symptoms?**

Peripheral paresthesias, Chvostek's sign, Trousseau's sign, tetany, seizures and mental status changes.

☐☐ **What is the most serious consequence of hypocalcemia?**

Laryngeal spasm.

☐☐ **T/F: Femoral vein catheters have the highest infection rates and should not be used routinely.**

False.

HEENT PEARLS

Nature, time and patience are the three great physicians.
Bulgarian proverb

❑❑ **What is the most common complication of outpatient ENT surgery?**

Postoperative hemorrhage.

❑❑ **When should patients be asked to discontinue aspirin or aspirin-containing drugs before ENT surgery?**

At least 1 week prior to elective surgery.

❑❑ **Branchial cleft cysts arise from which branchial clefts?**

The second and third.

❑❑ **What is the most common cause of epiglottitis?**

Haemophilus influenza.

❑❑ **What is the most common local complaint in adults with acute epiglottitis?**

Dysphagia.

❑❑ **What are the most common causes of grunting in children?**

Pneumonia, asthma and bronchiolitis.

❑❑ **What is the most common cause of sialoadenitis?**

Mumps.

❑❑ **What is the most common site of bleeding in posterior epistaxis?**

The lateral nasal branch of the sphenopalatine artery.

❑❑ **A 47 year old female presents to the ED with a complaint of excruciating waxing and waning, electric shock type pain in the right cheek. What is the most likely diagnosis?**

Tic douloureux.

❑❑ **What is the treatment of choice for hematomas of the pinna?**

Aspiration followed by splinting.

❑❑ **What organism is most frequently associated with auricular perichondritis?**

Pseudomonas aeruginosa.

❑❑ **Why are children more susceptible to acute otitis media?**

They have shorter, more horizontal eustachian tubes that prevent adequate drainage and allow aspiration of nasopharyngeal bacteria into the middle ear, particularly with upper respiratory tract infections.

❏❏ **What is the most reliable technique for culturing the causative organism in acute otitis media?**

Tympanocentesis.

❏❏ **What is the most common location for a cystic hygroma?**

The posterior triangle of the neck.

❏❏ **Which autosomal dominant syndrome is characterized by multiple osteomas of the mandible and maxilla, epidermoid cysts, adenomatous colonic polyps and intestinal desmoid tumors?**

Gardner's syndrome.

❏❏ **What is Kiesselbach's area?**

The confluence of septal branches of the superior labial branch of the facial artery, greater palatine artery, sphenopalatine artery and the anterior ethmoidal artery.

❏❏ **What syndrome is characterized by unilateral facial paralysis, a fissured tongue and facial swelling?**

Melkersson-Rosenthal Syndrome.

T/F: Non-epithelial cancers are the most prevalent malignancies in carcinoma of the larynx.

False. Squamous cell carcinoma is the most common (95 to 98%).

T/F: Cancers of the buccal mucosa arise more frequently from pre-existing leukoplakia than other oral cancers.

True.

❏❏ **Mistaken as tumors of the maxilla and mandible, these non-tender, hard, rounded swellings start early in life but are commonly unrecognized until mid-life. In the maxilla, they are located in the midline, posterior hard palate, in the mandible, on the lingual surface near the premolars. What are these lesions?**

Torus palatinus and torus mandibularis (exostoses of the bone).

❏❏ **What is the advantage of using laser for surgery?**

Laser is precise and nontraumatic to healthy tissue and produces less postoperative edema and pain.

❏❏ **What risk do lasers pose to patients and healthcare providers?**

Damage to eyes and skin, electrical shock, fire, explosion and production of noxious fumes.

❏❏ **What is the most common complication of otitis media with extension of infection to the temporal bone?**

Labyrinthitis.

❏❏ **What is the most common pathway for spread of infection due to chronic otitis media?**

Extension by bony erosion.

❏❏ Otosclerosis accounts for what percentage of conductive hearing loss?

1%.

❏❏ Third arch derivatives are innervated by which cranial nerve?

IX (glossopharyngeal).

❏❏ What drug might you give prior to extubation to decrease the risk of laryngospasm?

Lidocane.

❏❏ What is the initial treatment of laryngospasm?

Remove the stimulus, jaw-thrust and positive pressure ventilation with 100% oxygen.

❏❏ A patient presents with a foul smelling painless otorrhea and sensorineural hearing loss. What is the most likely diagnosis?

Syphilitic otitis media.

❏❏ What are the most likely pathogens in acute mastoiditis?

Streptococcus pneumonia, Streptococcus pyogenes and Staphylococcus aureus.

❏❏ An elderly female presents with headaches, stiffness in her joints, jaw/facial pain and visual loss. What is the most likely diagnosis?

Temporal arteritis (giant cell arteritis).

❏❏ A 42 year old female presents with dull right ear and jaw pain and a burning sensation in the roof of her mouth. She also hears a popping sound when she opens and closes her mouth. Physical examination reveals tenderness of the temperomandibular joint capsule. What is the most likely diagnosis?

TMJ syndrome.

❏❏ What is trench mouth (Vincent's disease)?

Acute necrotizing ulcerative gingivitis.

❏❏ What is the causative organism in trench mouth?

Treponema vincentii.

❏❏ What is the most common site of distant metastases from SCC of the head and neck?

The lung (80%).

❏❏ What is the most common neoplasm of the nasopharynx in children?

Lymphoma.

❏❏ What is the most common etiology of serious reactions to local anesthetics?

Inadvertent intravascular injection.

❏❏ What is the etiology of sleep apnea?

Two-thirds are primarily obstructive in origin and compounded by obesity. Neurologic dysfunction, including primary central nervous system dysfunction and behavioral disorders are present in nearly one-half of patients.

❑❑ **A 3 year old male presents with a unilateral purulent rhinorrhea. What is the most likely diagnosis?**

A nasal foreign body.

❑❑ **At what age does laryngotracheobronchitis (croup) typically occur?**

6 months to 6 years but usually in children under the age of 3.

❑❑ **What infection is associated with the lumpy jaw syndrome?**

Actinomycosis.

❑❑ **T/F: Adjuvant chemotherapy improves outcome for patients with head and neck neoplasms.**

False.

❑❑ **What are the most important risk factors for rhinocerebral mucormycosis?**

Neutropenia and diabetic ketoacidosis.

❑❑ **T/F: Surgical debridement is required for effective management of rhinocerebral mucormycosis.**

True.

❑❑ **A 4 year old female presents with ear pain and fluid-filled blisters on the tympanic membrane. What is the most likely diagnosis?**

Bullous myringitis.

❑❑ **A 19 year old male returns to the emergency department with fever, nausea, vomiting and hypotension two days after nasal packing was placed for an anterior nosebleed. What is the most likely diagnosis?**

Toxic shock syndrome.

❑❑ **What is the most frequent cause of hearing loss?**

Cerumen impaction.

❑❑ **Which muscles are involved in eustachian tube opening?**

The tensor veli palatini acting synergistically with the levator veli palatini.

❑❑ **What organisms are most commonly associated with angular cheilitis?**

Candida albicans and staphylococcus and streptococcus species.

❑❑ **What is the etiology of preauricular sinus tracts?**

Improper fusion of the first and second branchial arches.

❏❏ A 45 year old female complains of persistent hoarseness after exploration for a parathyroid adenoma. Laryngoscopy reveals that the vocal cords meet to the right of the midline. What is the diagnosis?

Injury to the right recurrent laryngeal nerve.

❏❏ What is the most common branchial anomaly?

A branchial cyst.

❏❏ Which branchial cleft lesion most often courses medially to the facial nerve?

A type w branchial cleft fistula.

❏❏ The most common glomus tumor in the head region is associated with what structure?

The jugular bulb.

❏❏ What is the diagnostic test of choice for acoustic neuromas?

An MRI with gadolinium.

❏❏ What anatomical nasal structure is the greatest contributor to total airway resistance?

The nasal valve.

❏❏ What is the most common site of cancer in the oral cavity?

The lip.

❏❏ What are the common causes of tympanic membrane perforation?

Blast injuries, foreign bodies, lightning strikes, otitis media and temporal bone fractures.

❏❏ What are the most frequent causes of auricular perichondritis?

Ear-piercing, acupuncture and trauma.

❏❏ T/F: Dermoid cysts arise along lines of embryologic fusion in the floor of the mouth.

True.

❏❏ Peritonsillar abscesses are most common in what age group?

Adolescents and young adults.

❏❏ What local sign is most frequently associated with a peritonsillar abscess?

Unilateral swelling of the soft palate.

❏❏ What is Lemierre's syndrome?

Septic thrombophlebitis of the internal jugular vein and septic pulmonary emboli associated with anaerobic oropharyngeal infection.

❏❏ What complication is associated with bilateral recurrent laryngeal nerve injury?

Closure of the glottis after extubation, a true emergency.

❐❐ **What contiguous infections are often associated with brain abscesses?**

Sinusitis and otitis.

❐❐ **What is the most important risk factor for malignant external otitis?**

Diabetes mellitus.

❐❐ **What is the most characteristic physical finding associated with malignant external otitis?**

Granulation tissue in the external auditory canal.

❐❐ **What structure drains into the inferior meatus of the nose?**

The nasolacrimal duct.

❐❐ **A 24 year old female presents with a fever, headache and malaise. Her physical examination is unremarkable except for a raised lesion on her nasal dorsum with an advancing border. The skin is tense, hot, tender and dark red. What is the most likely diagnosis?**

Erysipelas.

❐❐ **A baseball player presents 4 days after sustaining blunt trauma to his nose and complains of right sided nasal obstruction. Physical examination reveals a mildly displaced nasal dorsum and a reddish blue fluctuant swelling beneath the mucosa of his septum. What is the most likely diagnosis?**

A septal hematoma.

❐❐ **What factors predispose to sinus mucocele formation?**

Chronic infection, trauma, osteoma and allergies.

❐❐ **What is the most common cause of nasal obstruction in all age groups?**

Acute viral rhinitis (the common cold).

❐❐ **What is the sensory innervation of the nose?**

V_1 (nasociliary, external nasal and infratrochlear nerves) and V_2 (infraorbital nerve).

❐❐ **What structures drain into the middle meatus?**

The anterior ethmoid, maxillary and frontal sinuses.

❐❐ **What are the most common findings associated with orbital floor fractures?**

Diplopia and an inferiorly displaced globe.

❐❐ **A 10 year old female presents for evaluation of hearing loss and renal abnormalities. You note webbing of her neck, low set ears, large ear lobes and short stature. What chromosomal abnormality should you suspect?**

XO (Turner's syndrome).

❐❐ **What is the most common motor cranial nerve damaged in head trauma?**

CN VII (facial nerve).

❑❑ **Glomus tumors are composed of what type of cell?**

Paraganglion cells.

❑❑ **What virus has a strong association with nasopharyngeal carcinoma (NPC)?**

Epstein-Barr virus (EBV).

❑❑ **What are the boundaries for a radical neck dissection?**

The mandible superiorly, clavicle inferiorly, anterior border of the trapezius muscle posteriorly, the midline in the upper neck and the strap muscles in the lower neck.

❑❑ **What is the difference between a radical neck dissection and a modified radical neck dissection?**

In a radical neck dissection, the sternocleidomastoid muscle, lymph nodes and investing fascia, internal jugular vein, submandibular gland and spinal accessory nerve (CN X) are removed in an en bloc resection. With a modified radical neck dissection, the spinal accessory nerve and the internal jugular vein are spared.

❑❑ **Which views on routine x-ray are most sensitive in the diagnosis of acute infection of the paranasal sinuses?**

The Caldwell and Waters views.

❑❑ **Which intrinsic muscle of the tongue is not innervated by CN XII (hypoglossal nerve)?**

The palatoglossus muscle.

❑❑ **What is the most common tumor of the juvenile larynx?**

Laryngeal papilloma.

❑❑ **What major artery is contained within the space of the cavernous sinus?**

The internal carotid artery.

❑❑ **What diagnosis should be considered when an adolescent male presents with nasal obstruction and epistaxis?**

Juvenile nasopharyngeal angiofibroma.

❑❑ **What is the innervation of the larynx?**

The superior laryngeal nerve supplies sensation above the vocal cords and motor function of the cricothyroid muscle. The recurrent laryngeal nerve provides innervation to all remaining intrinsic laryngeal muscles and sensation below the vocal cords.

❑❑ **What is the differential diagnosis of partial airway obstruction in children?**

Extrinsic pathology: peritonsillar abscess, Ludwig's angina, cystic hygroma, vascular abnormalities and neoplasms. Intrinsic pathology: epiglottitis, croup, subglottic stenosis, vocal cord paralysis and laryngeal stricture anomalies.

❑❑ **What factors predispose patients to development of head and neck cancer?**

History of chronic cigarette smoking, alcohol use and advanced age.

❏❏ **What is the most common presenting symptom of patients with an acoustic neuroma?**

Hearing loss. Tinnitus is the second most common.

❏❏ **Acoustic neuromas are actually tumors of what structure?**

They are schwannomas derived from the superior division of the vestibular nerve.

❏❏ **What infection precedes acute orbital cellulitis in the majority of cases?**

Acute sinusitis.

❏❏ **What local signs are strongly suggestive of orbital cellulitis?**

Proptosis and pain.

❏❏ **What plain radiographic views are most helpful in visualizing facial fractures?**

The Water's view, a modified basal view of the skull and panorex.

❏❏ **What is a Le Fort II fracture?**

A facial fracture involving the facial aspects of the maxillae extending to the nasal and ethmoid bones, the maxillary sinuses, infraorbital rims bilaterally and across the nasal bridge. This is also called a pyramidal fracture.

❏❏ **What is the most common presenting symptom of NPC?**

Painless, unilateral, metastatic cervical lymphadenopathy.

❏❏ **What is the most effective primary treatment of NPC?**

Chemoradiotherapy using 5-fluorouracil/cisplatin and 66 to 70 Gy of radiation.

❏❏ **What is the primary cause of lip cancer?**

Long-term ultraviolet light exposure.

❏❏ **What is the most common type of mandible fracture?**

Alveolar.

❏❏ **What are the clinical signs of a basilar skull fracture?**

Blood behind the tympanic membrane, periorbital ecchymosis (raccoon eyes) and ecchymosis behind the ear (battle sign).

❏❏ **What is the etiology of thyroglossal duct cysts?**

Failure of obliteration of the midline pharyngeal diverticulum during thyroid descent.

❏❏ **What is the best radiographic view to visualize a zygomatic arch fracture?**

A modified basal view of the skull (also known as a jug-handle, submentaloccipital or submental-vertical view).

❏❏ **What is considered the supraglottic portion of the larynx?**

The laryngeal surface of the epiglottis, aryepiglottic folds, laryngeal surfaces of the arytenoids, the false or ventricular folds and the ventricles.

❑❑ **How many minor salivary glands are found within the submucosal plane of the oral cavity in the normal individual?**

Between 700 and 1,000.

❑❑ **What percentage of minor salivary gland tumors are malignant?**

75%.

❑❑ **What is the most common malignant tumor in the submandibular or minor salivary glands?**

Adenoid cystic carcinoma or cylindroma.

❑❑ **What mandibular malignancy is associated with a soap-bubble radiographic appearance?**

An ameloblastoma.

❑❑ **Non-epidermoid cancers make up what percentage of oral cavity cancers?**

Less than 10%.

❑❑ **What is the inheritance pattern of familial paraganglionomas?**

Autosomal dominant with variable penetrance.

❑❑ **What is the lymphatic drainage from the oral vestibule?**

The submental and submandibular lymph nodes.

❑❑ **What is the lymphatic drainage from the anterior third of the tongue?**

The submandibular, subdigastric and internal jugular nodes.

❑❑ **A singer has noted loss of her upper singing register 6 months after thyroid surgery. On examination, her right vocal cord assumes an intermediate position? What is the most likely diagnosis?**

A combined injury of the superior and recurrent laryngeal nerve.

❑❑ **What is the most common cause of bilateral vocal cord paralysis?**

Thyroidectomy.

❑❑ **What is the most common congenital laryngeal disorder?**

Laryngomalacia.

❑❑ **What is the most common origin of infection in patients with Ludwig's angina?**

A dental abscess.

❑❑ **What are the most common local findings in patients with Ludwig's angina?**

Edema of the floor of the mouth and tongue.

❏❏ What is the most common cause of death in Ludwig's angina?

Asphyxiation.

❏❏ What is the second most common benign tumor of the parotid gland?

A Warthin's tumor.

❏❏ A patient presents with a mobile, 2 cm right parotid mass. What is the most likely diagnosis?

A pleomorphic adenoma.

❏❏ What is the most common primary parotid gland malignancy?

Mucoepidermoid carcinoma.

❏❏ What are the major risk factors for development of oral cavity cancer?

Tobacco, alcohol, sunlight, poor dentition and occupational exposures such as isopropyl oils, sulfuric acid and nickel metallic ducts.

❏❏ What factors are associated with post-extubation croup?

A tight-fitting endotracheal tube, traumatic or repeated intubations, coughing while intubated, passive head repositioning, a previous history of post-extubation croup and prolonged intubation.

❏❏ A vertiginous patient undergoes cold calorics and develops a left beating nystagmus. Which ear is being stimulated?

The right (cold opposite, warm same).

❏❏ Which muscle is the sole abductor of the vocal cords?

The posterior cricoarytenoid.

❏❏ The cricothyroid muscle is innervated by what nerve?

The external branch of the superior laryngeal nerve.

❏❏ What is the innervation of the tensor tympani muscle?

The trigeminal nerve (V3).

❏❏ What is the most common pediatric salivary tumor?

A hemangioma.

❏❏ What is the most common benign tumor of the parotid gland?

A pleomorphic adenoma (benign mixed tumor).

❏❏ What are the symptoms of Meniere's disease?

Aural fullness, fluctuating hearing loss, tinnitus and vertigo.

❏❏ Referred ear pain from inflammation or cancer of the larynx/pharynx is via which combination of cranial nerves?

The trigeminal, glossopharyngeal and vagus nerves.

❏❏ **What is the most common salivary gland tumor?**

Pleomorphic adenoma.

❏❏ **What is the most feared complication of lateral pharyngeal space infections?**

Septic thrombophlebitis of the jugular vein.

❏❏ **What is Steven's Johnson Syndrome?**

Erythema multiforme in patients with additional findings of conjunctival, mouth and skin lesions, fever and leukopenia. The genitalia may also be involved.

❏❏ **What is the name of the submandibular gland duct and where does it exit within the mouth?**

Wharton's duct. It opens at the side of the tongue's frenulum behind the central mandibular incisors.

❏❏ **What is Horner's Syndrome?**

Exophthalmos, ptosis, miosis and anhidrosis.

❏❏ **What areas drain into the parotid lymph nodes?**

The temporal and postauricular scalp, pinna and the external auditory canal.

❏❏ **What is the most common presentation of a retropharyngeal abscess?**

Fever, stridor, dysphagia, refusal to eat, drooling and an opisthotonic position.

❏❏ **What is the most common organism associated with retropharyngeal abscesses?**

Beta-hemolytic streptococcus.

❏❏ **In a conductive hearing loss, to which ear does sound lateralize when using the Weber test?**

To the ear with the conductive hearing loss.

❏❏ **Infection at what site predisposes to cavernous sinus thrombosis?**

The orbit.

❏❏ **What are the most common local signs of cavernous sinus thrombosis?**

Bilateral proptosis and ophthalmoplegia.

❏❏ **What studies are most helpful in establishing the diagnosis of cavernous sinus thrombosis?**

CT and MRI.

❏❏ **T/F: Anticoagulant therapy decreases the mortality rate of cavernous sinus thrombosis.**

False.

❏❏ **What is the maximal amount of the lip (not involving the commissure) that can be closed primarily?**

One-third.

❑❑ **What are the primary lymphatics for the lateral lower lip?**

The ipsilateral submandibular lymph nodes.

❑❑ **What are the primary lymphatics for the upper lip?**

The ipsilateral submandibular and infra-auricular lymph nodes.

❑❑ **What type of repair is optimal for larger lip defects (up to 70% of the lip)?**

A Karapandzic flap.

❑❑ **What are the principal sites of lymphatic drainage from the oral cavity?**

Zones I, II and III (the submandibular, upper jugular and mid-jugular nodes).

❑❑ **What is the incidence of neck metastases in T1 oral cancer?**

20 to 30%.

❑❑ **What is the incidence of cervical metastases at the time of primary oropharyngeal carcinoma presentation?**

50 to 80%.

❑❑ **After squamous cell carcinoma, what is the next most common type of malignancy to occur in the oropharynx?**

Non-Hodgkin's lymphoma.

❑❑ **Why does glottic carcinoma have a relatively low risk of cervical metastases?**

There are few lymphatics underlying the true vocal cords.

❑❑ **What embryologic membranes limit the local spread of laryngeal carcinoma?**

The quadrangular membrane in the supraglottic larynx and the conus elasticus in the glottic and subglottic regions of the larynx.

❑❑ **What percentage of patients with advanced hypopharyngeal or cervical esophageal carcinoma have paratracheal (Zone VI) lymph node involvement?**

80%.

❑❑ **What is the lymphatic drainage of the hypopharynx?**

Zones II to IV (the upper, middle and lower jugular chain) and Zone VI (paratracheal).

❑❑ **Following a total pharyngoesophagectomy, what is the reconstructive procedure of choice?**

A gastric pull-up (transposition).

❑❑ **Why are hypopharyngeal and esophageal cancers prone to local recurrence?**

Extensive submucosal spread and skip lesions.

❑❑ **What are the Zone I neck lymph nodes?**

The submental and submandibular lymph nodes.

❑❑ **What is the diagnostic test of choice in evaluating a neck mass?**

Fine needle aspiration (FNA).

❑❑ **What is the incidence of perineural spread in adenoid cystic carcinoma?**

80%.

❑❑ **In which of the four major sinuses does cancer most frequently arise?**

The maxillary sinus.

❑❑ **Skull base chordomas arise from what embryonic precursor?**

The notochord.

❑❑ **What is the most common tumor of the parapharyngeal space?**

A deep lobe parotid tumor (pleomorphic adenoma).

❑❑ **Which muscles attach to the temporal bone?**

The posterior digastric, temporal, longus capitus and sternocleidomastoid muscles.

❑❑ **What is the blood supply to the middle ear and mastoid?**

The stylomastoid, deep auricular, middle meningeal and carotidotypmanic arteries.

❑❑ **What is the most common non-squamous cell carcinoma of the oral cavity?**

An adenoid cystic carcinoma of a minor salivary gland.

❑❑ **What anatomic factors are important in nasal airflow?**

The nasal septum, nasal valve, nasal vestibule and turbinates.

❑❑ **What are the components of the vidian nerve?**

The deep petrosal and greater superficial petrosal nerves.

❑❑ **Which paranasal sinuses are pneumatized at birth?**

The maxillary, ethmoid and sphenoid sinuses.

❑❑ **An injection of local anesthetic is made and almost immediately a seizure occurs. What is the most likely cause?**

Intravenous injection.

❑❑ **What symptoms usually suggest irritative or infiltrating disease of the upper aerodigestive tract?**

Dysphagia, odynophagia, referred otalgia and hoarseness.

❏❏ **The integrity of which laryngeal cartilage is essential in maintaining an airway?**

The cricoid cartilage.

❏❏ **What is the most definitive examination for identifying the site of a pharyngoesophageal injury?**

Rigid esophagoscopy.

❏❏ **What is the sensory innervation of the esophagus?**

The first through fifth thoracic sensory roots and the sympathetic nervous system.

❏❏ **How much mucous is produced by the nose?**

1 to 2 liters/day.

❏❏ **What is Waldeyer's ring?**

Lymphoid tissue surrounding the oropharyngeal inlet, specifically composed of the two pharyngeal tonsils, the adenoid and lingual tonsils. Lymphoid patches along the posterior pharyngeal wall are sometimes included.

❏❏ **What is the antibiotic of choice for parapharyngeal abscesses?**

Penicillin.

❏❏ **What are the surgical approaches to cancers of the oropharynx?**

Transoral, composite resection with mandibulectomy (Commando procedure), mandibulotomy and transhyoid/lateral pharyngotomy.

❏❏ **What structure separates the superficial (lateral) lobe of the parotid gland from the deep lobe?**

The facial nerve.

ESOPHAGUS, STOMACH, DUODENUM AND DIAPHRAGM PEARLS

Eat and drink measurely, and defy the mediciners.
Proverb

❑❑ **What is the blood supply to the esophagus?**

The cervical portion is supplied by the inferior thyroid arteries, the thoracic portion from the aorta and the abdominal portion from branches of the left gastric artery.

❑❑ **What is primary peristalsis?**

The propulsive wave that starts when a bolus is in the upper esophagus and forces the bolus toward the stomach. This is facilitated by relaxation of the lower esophageal sphincter (LES).

❑❑ **What is the treatment of choice for trichobezoars?**

Laparotomy, gastrotomy and operative removal.

❑❑ **What is the most common extranodal site of Non-Hodgkin's lymphoma?**

The stomach.

❑❑ **What are the main features of achalasia?**

Aperistalsis, incomplete relaxation of the LES during swallowing and increased resting LES pressure.

❑❑ **The phrenoesophageal ligament is a continuation of what abdominal structure?**

The transversalis fascia

❑❑ **T/F: Adenomatous gastric polyps are associated with gastric cancer.**

True.

❑❑ **What are the primary treatment options for achalasia?**

Pneumatic dilatation and (Heller's) esophagomyotomy.

❑❑ **What are the most common symptoms associated with diffuse esophageal spasm (DES)?**

Pain and dysphagia.

❑❑ **What are the diagnostic features of DES?**

Manometric demonstration of simultaneous, repetitive and occasionally prolonged pressure increases of considerable magnitude with a normal LES. Contrast studies show a corkscrew esophagus.

❏❏ **What are the complications of gastroesophageal reflux (GER)?**

Intractable heartburn, esophagitis, stenosis and shortening of the esophagus, Barrett's esophagus, motility disturbances, esophageal ulcer or bleeding and aspiration pneumonia.

❏❏ **What is Barrett's esophagus?**

The replacement of normal esophageal epithelium with columnar epithelium.

❏❏ **T/F: Correction of GER causes regression of Barrett's esophagus.**

False.

❏❏ **What is the most common presentation of a foramen of Bochdalek hernia?**

Respiratory distress shortly after birth.

❏❏ **What is a foramen of Morgagni hernia?**

An anterior herniation located at the sternocostal junction on either side of the xiphoid process.

❏❏ **What is the most common diverticulum of the esophagus and where is it located?**

A Zenker's diverticulum, located at the pharyngoesophageal junction. Typically it is located in the posterior midline between the oblique fibers of the inferior pharyngeal constrictors, just above the transverse fibers of the cricopharyngeus.

❏❏ **What is the most common cause of traction diverticula?**

Chronic, inflamed and granulomatous parabronchial lymph nodes

❏❏ **What are the treatment options for a patient with a Zenker's diverticulum?**

Cricopharyngeal myotomy alone or myotomy with diverticulectomy or diverticulopexy.

❏❏ **What is the most common benign tumor of the esophagus?**

A leiomyoma.

❏❏ **What is diaphragmatic eventration?**

Complete or partial unilateral elevation of the diaphragm without a localized defect.

❏❏ **T/F: Acute diaphragmatic injuries are best managed transthoracically.**

False.

❏❏ **What is the most common type of gastric volvulus?**

Organoaxial volvulus.

❏❏ **What is Plummer-Vinson syndrome?**

Atrophic oral mucosa, spoon-shaped fingers, brittle nails, iron deficiency anemia and dysphagia, often due to a fibrous esophageal web.

❑❑ **What is a Mallory-Weiss tear?**

A linear tear in the mucosa at the esophagogastric junction.

❑❑ **What is the best method of distinguishing malignant from benign gastric ulcers?**

Multiple biopsies.

❑❑ **T/F: The majority of patients with Mallory-Weiss syndrome require surgical repair.**

False.

❑❑ **What is Boerhaave's syndrome?**

Spontaneous rupture of the esophagus, usually just above the diaphragm, associated with an episode of forceful vomiting or retching.

❑❑ **What is the most common cause of esophageal perforation?**

Esophageal instrumentation.

❑❑ **What is the most common site of perforation of the esophagus?**

At the esophageal introitus, just proximal to the cricopharyngeus muscle.

❑❑ **What physical finding is associated with mediastinal emphysema?**

Hamman's sign (auscultation reveals precordial crackles that are synchronous with the heartbeat).

❑❑ **What is the best treatment for the majority of esophageal perforations?**

Surgical exploration, reinforced primary repair and drainage.

❑❑ **T/F: Caustic strictures of the esophagus are more commonly associated with acid ingestion than alkaline ingestion.**

False.

❑❑ **T/F: Esophagoscopy should be performed early after ingestion of a caustic agent.**

True. It is important to evaluate the extent of injury.

❑❑ **What is the most common inflammatory lesion of the esophagus?**

Moniliasis.

❑❑ **How many anastomoses are required when using the colon as an esophageal substitute?**

Three.

❑❑ **What manometric findings are associated with scleroderma?**

Normal esophageal peristalsis in the proximal striated muscle and aperistalsis of the distal smooth muscle. The LES decreases in pressure as the disease progresses.

❑❑ **What are the pathophysiologic mechanisms for GER?**

A defective LES, ineffective esophageal clearance and an abnormal gastric reservoir.

❐❐ **What is the most sensitive test for detection of GER?**

24-hour pH monitoring.

❐❐ **What is the most common malignant tumor of the esophagus?**

Squamous cell carcinoma.

❐❐ **T/F: It is important to have a wide surgical margin of resection during esophagectomy, even when margins are grossly negative.**

True. Esophageal carcinoma is prone to submucosal spread and skip lesions.

❐❐ **What are the most common symptoms of esophageal cancer?**

Progressive dysphagia and weight loss.

❐❐ **Esophageal reconstruction with a gastric pull-up is based on what blood supply?**

The right gastroepiploic artery is the primary blood supply with additional blood supply from the right gastric artery. The left gastroepiploic, left gastric and short gastric arteries are routinely divided.

❐❐ **How do nicotine, alcohol and chocolate affect the LES?**

They all decrease LES pressure.

❐❐ **T/F: The Bernstein test should be performed prior to antireflux surgery.**

True.

❐❐ **What are the late complications of corrosive burns of the esophagus?**

Stricture, GER and malignancy.

❐❐ **T/F: The operative mortality of esophagectomy is less than 10%.**

True.

❐❐ **T/F: Involvement of non-regional lymph nodes in esophageal carcinoma is considered metastatic disease.**

True.

❐❐ **What are the most important determinants of survival after resection of an esophageal carcinoma?**

Depth of invasion, the presence or absence of lymph node metastases and the presence or absence of distant metastases.

❐❐ **Tumor invasion of an adjacent structure suggests what T descriptor and tumor stage?**

T4, Stage III.

❐❐ **What are the most common sites of visceral metastases for esophageal cancer?**

The liver and lungs.

❏❏ **What is the main blood supply of the colonic conduit when using an isoperistaltic left colon for esophageal replacement?**

The ascending branch of the left colic artery.

❏❏ **What is the best palliative treatment for stage IV esophageal cancer?**

Endoluminal stenting.

❏❏ **What is the 5-year survival rate for a completely resected T1N0 adenocarcinoma of the esophagus?**

60%.

❏❏ **In what scenario may initial nonoperative management of an esophageal perforation be appropriate?**

With a contained localized perforation that is free of mediastinal or pleural contamination in a patient without clinical signs or symptoms of sepsis and where the esophagus distal to the site of perforation is not obstructed.

❏❏ **T/F: A limited distal esophagogastrectomy is appropriate in the management of an early carcinoma, arising in a segment of Barrett's changes and extending from 24 to 40 cm.**

False.

❏❏ **What are the complications of a prolonged chylous leak?**

Lymphopenia, immunosuppression, malnutrition, loss of proteins, fats and fat soluble vitamins, dehydration and electrolyte loss.

❏❏ **What are the major risk factors for development of an esophageal squamous cell carcinoma in North America?**

Nicotine and alcohol.

❏❏ **What are the indications for an anti-reflux procedure in a patient with Barrett's esophagus without dysplasia?**

Poor medical control of symptoms or complications such as stricture, ulceration or perforation.

❏❏ **T/F: There is no need for continued surveillance endoscopies in a patient with Barrett's esophagus who has undergone an effective anti-reflux procedure.**

False.

❏❏ **T/F: Stage for stage, the survival of patients with esophageal cancer treated with combined chemotherapy and radiation therapy has been clearly shown to be inferior to surgical resection or trimodality therapy.**

False.

❏❏ **What is the main risk of radiation therapy for an unresectable mid-esophageal cancer that involves the left main stem bronchus?**

The creation of a bronchoesophageal fistula.

❏❏ T/F: Induction radiation therapy followed by surgery improves the survival of esophageal cancer over that obtained by surgery alone.

False.

❏❏ What are the characteristics of eosinophilic gastroenteritis?

Polypoid or diffuse eosinophilic infiltration of the antrum.

❏❏ T/F: Combination chemoradiotherapy has been shown to be superior to radiation therapy alone in the treatment of non-metastatic esophageal cancer.

True.

❏❏ T/F: Combination induction chemotherapy and radiation followed by surgery appears to improve 5-year survival compared to surgery alone in resectable esophageal cancer.

True.

❏❏ What are the common postoperative complications of esophagectomy?

Pneumonia, anastomotic leak, anastomotic stricture, chylothorax, functional gastric outlet obstruction and reflux.

❏❏ What is the major blood supply to the foregut and stomach?

The celiac artery.

❏❏ What major structures support the stomach?

The gastrocolic, gastrosplenic and gastrophrenic ligaments.

❏❏ T/F: Bethanecol increases LES pressure.

True.

❏❏ What part of the autonomic nervous system is responsible for the sensation of stomach pain?

Afferent fibers of the sympathetic nervous system.

❏❏ What are the major types of secreting cells of the stomach mucosa?

Superficial epithelial, parietal, chief and gastrin cells.

❏❏ What is the most important stimulant for gastrin release?

A meal.

❏❏ T/F: The hepatic branch of the anterior vagus in also known as the anterior nerve of Latarjet.

False.

❏❏ What is the effect of somatostatin on gastrin secretion?

It is inhibitory.

❏❏ What membrane-bound protein is ultimately responsible for acid secretion?

The parietal cell proton pump.

❏❏ **What is involved in the Belsey procedure?**

Two layers of plicating sutures placed between the gastric fundus and the lower esophagus with subsequent creation of a 280° anterior gastric wrap and posterior approximation of the crura.

❏❏ **What is the most important physiologic function of pepsin?**

It initiates protein digestion.

❏❏ **What is the importance of gastric bicarbonate production?**

It is the major protective mechanism for the mucosal surface.

❏❏ **What events affect the rate of gastric blood flow?**

Vagal stimulation, calcitonin gene-related peptide and prostaglandin E2.

❏❏ **What is receptive relaxation?**

Relaxation of the proximal stomach to accommodate the increases in volume caused by a meal.

❏❏ **T/F: The Hill procedure can be performed through an abdominal or thoracic approach.**

False.

❏❏ **What are the most common complications of type II hiatal hernias?**

Occult gastrointestintal bleeding, ulceration in the herniated portion of the stomach and gastric volvulus.

❏❏ **What is the largest size solid food particle that can pass through the pylorus?**

Usually, no more than 1 mm.

❏❏ **What is the most common malignant tumor of the duodenum?**

Adenocarcinoma.

❏❏ **How fast does gastric epithelium regenerate?**

Every 2 to 3 days.

❏❏ **A 40 year old female presents with dysphagia, regurgitation and chest pain. Esophageal findings include abnormal relaxation of the LES. What is the most likely diagnosis?**

Vigorous achalasia.

❏❏ **What is epithelial restitution?**

During stress, significant disruption of the mucosal surface can occur. However, if the damage is superficial, it can be repaired in a matter of minutes. Viable cells flatten out and cover denuded areas.

❏❏ **T/F: The gastric mucosa is hydrophobic.**

True.

❏❏ **What is the first line of defense of the gastric mucosa?**

The bicarbonate-rich fluid produced by gastric surface epithelial cells.

❏❏ What are Cushing's and Curling's ulcers?

A Cushing's ulcer is acute gastritis or peptic ulcer disease that occurs as a result of central nervous system trauma or disease. A Curling's ulcer is a similar lesion observed after a significant burn injury.

❏❏ What are the major predisposing factors for stress gastritis?

Any event that potentially disrupts splanchnic perfusion. It has been observed after multi-system trauma, shock, sepsis, ARDS and prolonged surgery.

❏❏ What is the diagnostic test of choice for stomach ulcers?

Esophagogastroduodenoscopy (EGD).

❏❏ What stomach ulcer complications require surgical intervention?

Perforation, hemorrhage, obstruction and failure of medical treatment.

❏❏ What percentage of patients with an upper gastrointestinal (UGI) hemorrhage will stop bleeding without the need for surgical intervention?

Over 80%.

❏❏ What is the endoscopic treatment for a bleeding gastric ulcer?

Thermal, electric or laser coagulation. Injection of substances such as epinephrine or absolute alcohol may also stop active bleeding.

❏❏ What is the most common location of a stomach ulcer?

The lesser curvature, near the incisura angularis.

❏❏ What effects do non-steroidal anti-inflammatory drugs (NSAIDs) have on the stomach mucosa?

NSAIDs inhibit gastric mucosal cyclooxygenase and, thus, inhibit prostaglandin synthesis. The absence of prostaglandins weakens mucosal defenses and predisposes to ulcer formation.

❏❏ Which cranial nerves must be intact for successful treatment of a Zenker's diverticulum?

V, VII, X, XI and XII.

❏❏ What is the most sensitive diagnostic test for Helicobacter pylori?

Giemsa and Warthin-Starry stains. The urease breathing test is also very reliable but is available only in institutions with mass spectrophotometric capability.

❏❏ What are the most commonly prescribed agents for the treatment of gastric ulcer with confirmed Helicobacter pylori infection?

Bismuth subsalicylate, tetracycline and metronidazole.

❏❏ What endoscopic features of stomach ulcers suggest malignancy?

Presence of an exophytic mass, disrupted mucosal folds, a necrotic ulcer crater, stepwise depression and bleeding from the edge of the ulcer crater.

❑❑ **What are the most commonly prescribed agents for the treatment of gastric ulcer?**

H2-blockers.

❑❑ **T/F: Cervical esophageal dysphagia occurs in patients with Paterson-Kelley syndrome.**

True.

❑❑ **What is the procedure of choice for a Type I benign gastric ulcer?**

A Billroth I anastomosis.

❑❑ **What is the definition of a giant gastric ulcer?**

An ulcer with a diameter of 3 cm or greater.

❑❑ **What are the indications for emergent surgical treatment of gastric ulcers?**

Uncontrollable hemorrhage, rebleeding during the course of successful medical therapy and perforation.

❑❑ **What is the major risk factor for the development of a duodenal ulcer?**

Cigarette smoking.

❑❑ **What is the effect of diet on the rate of duodenal ulcer healing?**

None. (The role of alcohol and caffeine is unsettled and probably minimal.)

❑❑ **What is the maximal gastric acid output in normal men?**

Approximately 20 mEq/h.

❑❑ **T/F: Patients with a duodenal ulcer have an increased basal acid output.**

True.

❑❑ **What is the most common site of duodenal ulceration?**

The first portion of the duodenum.

❑❑ **What is the risk of recurrent ulceration after successful medical treatment of a duodenal ulcer with H2-blockers?**

Greater than 50% within 1 year.

❑❑ **What medications can be affected by co-administration of H2-blockers?**

Coumadin, phenytoin, diazepam, propranolol and theophylline.

❑❑ **What is the drug of choice for the treatment of a duodenal ulcer in pregnant women?**

Sucralfate.

❑❑ **What is the effect of vagotomy on gastric acid output?**

It reduces acid secretion by about 80% in the immediate postoperative period and diminishes parietal cell responsiveness to gastrin and histamine.

❏❏ **T/F: Emptying of solid food is affected by vagotomy.**

False.

❏❏ **What is the leading cause of death associated with peptic ulcer?**

Hemorrhage.

❏❏ **What is the surgical treatment of choice for a patient with an actively bleeding ulcer?**

Direct ligation of the bleeding vessel within the ulcer base followed by an acid reducing procedure.

❏❏ **What are the criteria for definitive versus delayed repair of a perforated ulcer?**

If there has been no preoperative shock or life-threatening coexisting medical illness and the perforation has been present for less than 48 hours, a definitive ulcer operation may be performed. If these criteria are not met, immediate simple omental patching is usually safer.

❏❏ **What signs and symptoms are associated with alkaline reflux gastritis?**

Postprandial epigastric pain, nausea, vomiting, reflux of bile into the stomach and histologic evidence of gastritis.

❏❏ **What is the most common symptom of progression of gastric cancer?**

Pain.

❏❏ **What is the best diagnostic test for gastric cancer?**

Fiberoptic endoscopy and biopsy.

❏❏ **What is the histologic appearance of the diffuse form of gastric carcinoma?**

Sheets of loosely adherent cells.

❏❏ **T/F: Surgery offers the only realistic chance of long-term survival for gastric cancer.**

True.

❏❏ **At what age do most gastric lymphomas occur?**

In the sixth and seventh decades of life.

❏❏ **What is the first step in the treatment of gastric lymphoma?**

Gastric resection.

❏❏ **What is the most common sarcoma of the stomach?**

Leiomyosarcoma.

❏❏ **Why are the symptoms of GER exacerbated in the evening?**

In the absence of food, the gastric environment is predominately acid and pepsin. Delayed gastric clearance during rest and decreased generation of saliva increases symptoms.

❏❏ **What LES pressure is diagnostic of resting GER?**

Less than 6 mm Hg.

❏❏ **What are the surgical indications for anti-reflux procedures?**

Patients refractory to medical therapy with persistent endoscopic evidence of esophagitis, esophageal stricture, Barrett's changes, radiographic evidence of recurrent aspiration pneumonia and a mechanically incompetent LES.

❏❏ **What magnitude of increased risk of esophageal adenocarcinoma is present in patients with Barrett's esophagus?**

Approximately 30% of patients with Barret's esophagus will ultimately develop adenocarcinoma

❏❏ **What is the most common site of esophageal perforation in Boerhaave's syndrome?**

The left posterolateral esophagus, 3-5 cm above the gastroesophageal (GE) junction.

❏❏ **What types of oxyntic glands are found in each region of the stomach?**

The isthmus contains mucous and parietal cells, the neck contains predominately parietal cells and the base contains chief cells.

❏❏ **T/F: The left gastroepiploic artery is very effective in maintaining gastric viability after subtotal gastrectomy in the absence of other vasculature.**

True.

❏❏ **What is the most common predisposing factor for stress gastritis in the critical care setting?**

Decreased gastric mucosal blood flow due to inadequate perfusion.

❏❏ **What are relative contraindications to parietal cell vagotomy?**

Prepyloric ulcers, gastric outlet obstruction, ulcerogenic medications that cannot be discontinued and cigarette smoking.

❏❏ **What is meant by a highly selective vagotomy?**

Division of individual branches of the nerve of Latarjet, preserving the crow's foot.

❏❏ **What is the most frequent complication of gastric ulcers?**

Perforation.

❏❏ **What is the primary anatomic location of parietal cells?**

In the gastric cardia.

❏❏ **What is the natural history of benign gastric ulcers?**

Most recovery uneventfully. However, the recurrence rate is as high as 70% within the first year.

❏❏ **T/F: All gastric polyps have a malignant potential.**

False.

❏❏ **What is linitus plastica?**

Thickening of the gastric wall with loss of rugae secondary to submucosal spread of adenocarcinoma.

❑❑ **T/F: Pernicious anemia increases the risk of developing gastric carcinoma.**

True.

❑❑ **In what region of the stomach does gastric carcinoma most frequently occur?**

Equally between the proximal and distal regions.

❑❑ **How often is metastatic disease present on initial presentation of gastric carcinoma?**

15%.

❑❑ **How extensive should surgical margins be to decrease the risk of recurrence of gastric carcinoma?**

5 to 6 cm.

❑❑ **What are the indications for surgery for patients with peptic ulcer disease (PUD)?**

Perforation, hemorrhage, obstruction and intractability.

❑❑ **What is the effect of cigarette smoking on preexisting PUD?**

It impairs ulcer healing and increases the rate of recurrence after healing.

❑❑ **How does cigarette smoking impair healing of peptic ulcers?**

It causes decreased prostaglandin generation, increased biliary reflux, increased gastric acid secretion and alterations in mucosal blood flow.

❑❑ **A 40 year old female presents with severe symptoms of PUD. What is the most common location of her ulcer?**

Within 2 to 3 cm of the pylorus, in the first portion of the duodenum.

❑❑ **What would be the most likely diagnosis for the above patient if the ulcer was found in the third or fourth portion of the duodenum?**

A gastrinoma.

❑❑ **How effective are H2-blockers for maintenance therapy for patients with PUD? What is the relapse rate?**

About 70% of patients are ulcer free endoscopically at 4 weeks of therapy and 80 to 90% are pain free at 8 weeks. There is a 15% relapse rate of ulceration despite adequate medical therapy.

❑❑ **What are the surgical options for patients with PUD?**

A highly selective vagotomy, vagotomy and pyloroplasty or vagotomy and antrectomy.

❑❑ **What anatomical landmarks identify the line of incision for an antrectomy?**

A line from the incisura angularis to a point on the greater curvature, midway between the pylorus and the GE junction.

❑❑ **How does a highly selective vagotomy (HSV) affect gastric emptying?**

HSV impairs receptive relaxation of the distal stomach, creating a pressure gradient with the duodenum and an increased rate of gastric emptying.

❑❑ **What is the leading cause of death in patients with PUD?**

Hemorrhage.

❑❑ **What are the endoscopic signs of recent ulcer bleeding?**

An adherent clot with oozing apparent from below, the vessel is visible in the ulcer base and sloughing in the ulcer base.

❑❑ **What symptoms characterize early dumping syndrome?**

Nausea, palpitations, epigastric pain and syncope. Late dumping occurs 1 to 3 hours after eating and is characterized by reactive hypoglycemia.

❑❑ **A 40 year old female with a history of PUD presents with sudden right scapular pain and severe abdominal pain. She is hemodynamically stable and otherwise healthy. Is an antiulcer procedure indicated at the time of exploration for perforation?**

Yes, given that the perforation is less than 24 hours old and is associated with a limited inflammatory response. If chronic disease is present, the patient is unstable or if the perforation is greater than 2 days old, omental patching of the ulcer with debridement of devitalized tissue is the appropriate option.

❑❑ **What surgical option is available for patients with severe dumping syndrome?**

Conversion of a Billroth I or II to a Roux-en-Y anastomosis.

❑❑ **What signs and symptoms are associated with alkaline gastric reflux?**

Postprandial epigastric pain with nausea and vomiting, gastric biliary reflux visualized endoscopically and histological changes consistent with alkaline gastritis.

APPENDIX AND INGUINAL HERNIA PEARLS

The patient suffered from chronic remunerative appendicitis.
Delbert H. Nickson

❏❏ **What is the most common position of the appendix found at autopsy?**

Retrocecal.

❏❏ **What are the typical locations of the appendix in order of frequency?**

Retrocecal-retrocolic, pelvic or descending, subcecal and ileocecal.

❏❏ **Where might the appendix be in a patient with dextrocardia?**

In the left lower quadrant.

❏❏ **What is the etiology of the classic periumbilical pain associated with appendicitis?**

Stretching of the inflamed appendiceal wall.

❏❏ **T/F: The appendix is a component of the secretory immune system.**

True.

❏❏ **Why is appendicitis rare in children under 2 years of age?**

The appendix has a wide lumen.

❏❏ **What is a pectineal hernia?**

The hernia sac enters through the femoral canal but perforates the pectineus muscle aponeurosis.

❏❏ **What is a Hesselbach hernia?**

This hernia passes into the pelvis lateral to the femoral vessels, below the inguinal ligament and the iliopubic tract.

❏❏ **What percentage of tumors of the appendix are carcinoid tumors?**

85%.

❏❏ **Where do the lymphatics of the appendix drain?**

The chain of nodes on the appendiceal, ileocolic and superior mesenteric arteries into the celiac lymph nodes.

❏❏ **Where is McBurney's point?**

Two-thirds the distance from the umbilicus on a line between the umbilicus and the anterosuperior iliac spine.

❏❏ **What is the average length of the appendix?**

9 cm, ranging from 2 to 20 cm.

❏❏ **The appendiceal artery is a branch of what artery?**

The ileocolic artery.

❏❏ **In classic appendicitis, where is the initial pain felt?**

In the periumbilical region.

❏❏ **What is Rovsing's sign?**

Pain in the right lower quadrant when checking for rebound tenderness in the left lower quadrant.

❏❏ **What is the psoas sign?**

Pain perceived during extension of the right hip.

❏❏ **What percentage of patients with appendicitis have an elevated white blood cell count?**

Two-thirds; only 4 to 5% will have a normal differential.

❏❏ **What are the causes of acute appendicitis?**

Hyperplasia of the submucosal lymphoid follicles (35%), fecal stasis or fecalith (4%), foreign bodies (4%) and strictures or tumors of the appendix or cecum (1%).

❏❏ **What age group has the maximal incidence of appendicitis?**

10 to 30 years old.

❏❏ **What area of the appendix most frequently shows evidence of gangrene and perforation?**

The midportion of the antimesenteric border.

❏❏ **What are the CT findings in acute appendicitis?**

A diameter greater than 6 mm, inflammatory changes in the mesentery and streaking of the fat.

❏❏ **What are the most common complications of appendectomy?**

Wound infection, intraabdominal abscess, fecal fistula, pyelophlebitis and intestinal obstruction.

❏❏ **What is the incidence of spontaneous abdominal hernia in the United States?**

5%.

❏❏ **What is the incidence of groin hernias in men?**

3%.

❏❏ **What percentage of premature male infants have an inguinal hernia?**

30%.

❑❑ **What is the ratio of the incidence of indirect to direct inguinal hernia?**

2:1.

❑❑ **What is the incidence of a patient processus vaginalis at birth?**

80%.

❑❑ **T/F: Femoral hernias are more common than inguinal hernias in women.**

False.

❑❑ **What superficial blood vessels are seen during an open inguinal hernia repair?**

The superficial epigastric, superficial circumflex iliac and the external pudendal arteries with their accompanying veins.

❑❑ **What is a strangulated hernia?**

One in which the vascularity of the protruded viscus is compromised.

❑❑ **What is the triangle of pain?**

The area between the iliopubic tract and the gonadal vessels, where the femoral nerve could be injured during laparoscopic hernia repairs.

❑❑ **T/F: Gangrene and perforation of the appendix occurs more commonly in children than in adults.**

True. This is usually due to a delay in diagnosis.

❑❑ **What is a pantaloon hernia?**

One that has a direct and an indirect component to the inguinal hernia.

❑❑ **What is a Maydl's hernia?**

When two successive loops of bowel enter the hernia sac and the loop inside the peritoneal cavity becomes gangrenous.

❑❑ **What is the superficial (external) inguinal ring?**

A triangular opening in the external oblique aponeurosis, slightly above and lateral to the pubic tubercle, transmitting the spermatic cord.

❑❑ **During surgery for presumed appendicitis, the appendix is found to be normal. However, the terminal ileum has an appearance consistent with Crohn's disease. Should appendectomy still be performed?**

Yes.

❑❑ **T/F: The iliopubic tract is a condensation of the transversalis fascia.**

True.

❑❑ **What nerve runs anterior to the spermatic cord in the inguinal canal?**

The ilioinguinal nerve.

❏❏ **What is the internal inguinal ring?**

An opening in the transversalis fascia.

❏❏ **Where is the internal inguinal ring located?**

At the mid-inguinal point, 1.25 cm above the midpoint of a line joining the symphysis pubis and the anterior superior iliac spine.

❏❏ **What are the boundaries of Hesselbach's triangle?**

The inguinal ligament inferiorly, the inferior epigastric artery laterally and the lateral border of the rectus sheath medially.

❏❏ **What are the boundaries of the femoral triangle?**

The femoral vein is the lateral boundary, the iliopubic tract lies anteriorly and medially and the pectineus fascia and superior pubic rami make up the posterior boundary.

❏❏ **What is the clinical difference between a femoral and an inguinal hernia?**

An inguinal hernia lies superior to the inguinal ligament, a femoral hernia is inferior. An inguinal hernia tends to expand medially and down into the scrotum, passing medial to the pubic tubercle, a femoral hernia expands laterally and then turns superiorly.

❏❏ **What is the difference between a direct and an indirect inguinal hernia?**

Indirect hernias originate lateral to the inferior epigastric vessels, whereas direct hernias originate medial to them.

❏❏ **What are the contents of the spermatic cord?**

The vas deferens and accompanying artery, the testicular artery and vein, lymphatics, autonomic nerves and fat.

❏❏ **What are the common causes for increased intraabdominal pressure that can result in a hernia?**

Chronic cough, chronic obstructive pulmonary disease, constipation (sometimes due to an underlying colorectal cancer), obstructive uropathy, massive ascites and pregnancy.

❏❏ **Which position is best to demonstrate a small reducible groin hernia?**

The upright position.

❏❏ **T/F: Repair of inguinal hernias in infants requires only high ligation of the hernial sac.**

True.

❏❏ **What is the differential diagnosis of an inguinal hernia?**

Hydrocele, lipoma of the cord, spermatocele, varicocele, undescended testis and tumor.

❏❏ **What is the differential diagnosis of a femoral hernia?**

Lymphadenopathy, lipoma, aneurysm or pseudoaneurysm of the femoral artery, lymphocele, hematoma or a psoas abscess.

❑❑ **What is the incidence of bowel obstruction in a hernia?**

5%.

❑❑ **What is a Shouldice repair?**

A variation of the Bassini repair with overlap of the transversalis plane and 4 lines of continuous sutures.

❑❑ **What is a McVay (Cooper ligament) repair?**

The transversus abdominus aponeurosis is approximated to Cooper's ligament.

❑❑ **When is a prosthetic mesh indicated for hernia repair?**

In patients with a weak posterior wall or patients with co-morbidities (e.g., malignancy, steroids, COPD and chronic cough).

❑❑ **What happens if the testicular artery is divided during a hernia repair?**

Usually, the testis survives due to collateral circulation. Only occasionally does it atrophy or undergo ischemic necrosis.

❑❑ **What are the signs of strangulation in a hernia?**

A painful, tense and non-reducible mass.

❑❑ **What is the single most important principle in hernia repair?**

Avoid tension.

❑❑ **What is the overall mortality rate in hernia repairs?**

Less than 1%.

❑❑ **What is the reported recurrence rate for the Bassini repair?**

5 to 20%.

❑❑ **What is the incidence of incisional hernias?**

3 to 5% of all abdominal operations. Male:Female is 1:2.

❑❑ **What are the predisposing factors for incisional hernias?**

Midline incisions, infections, emergency procedures, poor nutritional status, debilitating disorders (e.g., carcinoma, diabetes, ascites and cirrhosis), obesity, postoperative chest complications and presence of drainage tubes.

CARDIAC SURGERY PEARLS

No man really becomes a fool until he stops asking questions.
Charles Steinmetz

❏❏ **What congenital heart defects result in a left-to-right intracardiac shunt?**

An atrial septal defect (ASD), ventricular septal defect (VSD) and a patent ductus arteriosus (PDA).

❏❏ **What diagnostic tool is most likely to distinguish a secundum ASD from a primum ASD?**

ECG.

❏❏ **What are the branches of the subclavian artery?**

In order from proximal to distal, the vertebral artery, internal mammary artery, thyrocervical trunk and costocervical trunk.

❏❏ **What are the branches of the external carotid artery?**

In order from proximal to distal, the superior thyroid, ascending pharyngeal, lingual, facial, occipital, posterior auricular, internal maxillary and temporal arteries.

❏❏ **What are the boundaries of the triangle of Koch?**

The medial wall of the right atrium formed by the tendon of Todaro, the eustachian valve of the coronary sinus and the tricuspid annulus. The atrioventricular (AV) node is located subendocardially in this triangle.

❏❏ **What are the characteristics of the Scimitar syndrome?**

Hypoplasia of the right lung, anomalous venous return of the right lung to the inferior vena cava and an anomalous systemic arterial supply to the right lung.

❏❏ **What is a paradoxical embolus?**

A venous thrombus that goes through a right-to-left intracardiac shunt to the arterial side.

❏❏ **T/F: Osler's nodes are usually nodular and painful.**

True. In contrast, the macular Janeway lesions are painless.

❏❏ **What conditions, other than infective endocarditis, are associated with Osler's nodes?**

Nonbacterial thrombotic endocarditis, gonococcal infections and hemolytic anemia.

❏❏ **What is Bland, White and Garland syndrome?**

Sweating and irritability with feeding (considered an anginal equivalent in an infant) that occurs in infants with an anomalous origin of the left coronary artery from the pulmonary artery.

❏❏ **What is transient monocular blindness (amaurosis fugax)?**

A sudden blindness in one eye, described as if a shade were being pulled down. The blindness lasts minutes to hours and spontaneously resolves. This phenomenon is felt to be due to emboli to the terminal retinal arterioles from the carotid bifurcation.

❏❏ **What is the etiology of idiopathic hypertrophic subaortic stenosis (IHSS)?**

A hypertrophic myopathy of the left ventricular outflow tract.

❏❏ **What is the etiology of transposition of the great vessels?**

Abnormal development of the primitive bulbus cordis.

❏❏ **What congenital heart defects result in obstructive lesions and increased ventricular work?**

Pulmonic stenosis, aortic stenosis and coarctation of the aorta.

❏❏ **What is the appropriate therapy for a newborn with IHSS?**

Continuous infusion of prostaglandin E_1 (PGE_1), a low FIO_2 and a Norwood repair.

❏❏ **When do intracardiac shunts become physiologically important?**

When the pulmonary blood flow exceeds 1.5 to 2 times the systemic flow.

❏❏ **What concomitant cardiac defect is required for survival of patients with total anomalous pulmonary venous drainage?**

A patent ASD.

❏❏ **What is the etiology of the gracile habitus in children with a PDA or ASD?**

The shunt causes an increased blood flow through the pulmonary vasculature and decreased flow through the systemic vasculature, resulting in retardation of normal growth and development.

❏❏ **T/F: Squatting can increase systemic vascular resistance (SVR) and, thus, decrease right-to-left shunting.**

True.

❏❏ **What are cyanotic spells (tet spells)?**

Periodic episodes of unconsciousness related to cerebral hypoxia.

❏❏ **What radiologic finding is associated with the tetralogy of Fallot?**

A sabot-shaped heart.

❏❏ **What auscultatory finding is associated with a PDA?**

A widely split and fixed S2.

❏❏ **Which congenital heart defects are associated with congenital aortic stenosis?**

PDA, VSD, coarctation of the aorta and mitral valve defects.

❏❏ **What is the most reliable assessment of the severity of aortic stenosis?**

Measurement of peak systolic gradients.

❏❏ **What is the classic radiographic finding associated with coarctation of the aorta?**

Rib-notching.

❏❏ **T/F: ECG accurately determines the severity of obstruction in patients with pulmonic stenosis.**

True.

❏❏ **Right atrial enlargement is associated with which congenital heart defects?**

Ebstein's malformation, ASD and pulmonic stenosis.

❏❏ **What is the hallmark of congestive heart failure (CHF) in children?**

Hepatic enlargement.

❏❏ **What significant auscultatory finding occurs with mitral or tricuspid stenosis?**

A diastolic murmur.

❏❏ **What is the ethiology of bacterial endocarditis?**

Blood-borne bacteria that attach to damaged or abnormal heart valves or on the endocardium near anatomic defects.

❏❏ **What bacteremia-producing procedures increase the risk of developing bacterial endocarditis?**

Dental and oral procedures, those involving the respiratory mucosa, gastrointestinal procedures, genitourinary tract procedures and vaginal delivery.

❏❏ **What is the appropriate prophylaxis for these procedures?**

Depending upon the nature of the procedure, amoxicillin, ampicillin, gentamicin, clindamycin or a combination of these antibiotics are used.

❏❏ **Following a high-speed motor vehicle accident (MVA), evaluation reveals a widened mediastinum. What is the pathophysiology of the probable injury?**

The ligamentum arteriosum tethers the under surface of the aortic arch to the proximal left main pulmonary artery, at a point just distal to the left subclavian artery. Sudden deceleration causes shearing between the mobile aortic arch and the immobile descending aorta, resulting in aortic disruption.

❏❏ **When should a patient quit smoking to receive the most beneficial effect, prior to undergoing thoracic surgery?**

2 to 3 months prior to surgery.

❏❏ **What is the most common cause of ventricular aneurysms?**

A transmural myocardial infarction.

❏❏ **What are the most common causes of acute pericarditis?**

Idiopathic, infectious, neoplastic, radiation, uremia, myocardial infarction, autoimmune, rheumatologic, trauma, drugs and myxedema.

❐❐ **What triad of findings confirms the diagnosis of pericarditis?**

Chest pain, a pericardial friction rub and ECG abnormalities.

❐❐ **What organisms are most frequently implicated in endocarditis in intravenous drug abusers?**

Gram negative and fungal organisms.

❐❐ **What ECG changes are associated with pericarditis?**

ST elevation in all leads except V1 and VR. PR segment depression may also occur.

❐❐ **What is the most important regulator of coronary blood flow?**

Adenosine.

❐❐ **VSD accounts for what percentage of congenital heart defects?**

20 to 30%.

❐❐ **What are the four types of total anomalous pulmonary venous drainage?**

Supracardiac, intracardiac, infracardiac and mixed.

❐❐ **What is the most frequently reported bacterial isolate in patients with myocardial abscesses?**

Staphylococcus aureus.

❐❐ **What is mural endocarditis?**

Inflammation and disruption of the nonvalvular endocardial surface of the cardiac chambers.

❐❐ **What organism is most commonly associated with infection within the first month of pacemaker insertion?**

Staphylococcus aureus.

❐❐ **Which congenital heart defect is associated with Down's syndrome?**

An ostium primum ASD.

❐❐ **What are the typical features of Takayasu's arteritis?**

Early symptoms include fever, myalgias, arthralgias, weight loss and pain over inflamed vessels. Late symptoms are referable to occlusive changes and include transient ischemic attacks, stroke, arm fatigue, leg claudication and angina.

❐❐ **What are the laboratory markers for Takayasu's disease?**

An elevated erythrocyte sedimentation rate (ESR), leukocytosis and anemia of chronic disease.

❐❐ **What is the most common benign cardiac tumor?**

Myxoma.

❐❐ **What is the most common cardiac tumor in infancy?**

Rhabdomyoma.

❏❏ **What is the most common organism associated with endocarditis?**

Streptococcus viridans.

❏❏ **What is the major risk factor for prosthetic vascular graft infection?**

Location. The incidence of infection is 1 to 1.5% for aortoiliac grafts as opposed to 2 to 7% for femoropopliteal arterial grafts.

❏❏ **What is the most common cause of this infection?**

Contamination.

❏❏ **What criteria must be met to confirm the diagnosis of a line infection?**

A series of positive blood cultures and/or a positive line tip culture with greater than 15 colony forming units with the same organism.

❏❏ **T/F: Single lumen central venous catheters are less prone to infection.**

True.

❏❏ **What complications are associated with arterial catheterization?**

Thrombosis, infection, pseudoaneurysm and rupture.

❏❏ **What is the treatment for infected vascular catheters?**

Removal of the catheter and, possibly, antibiotic therapy.

❏❏ **What are the most common organisms involved with line infections?**

Staphylococcus epidermidis and Staphylococcus aureus.

❏❏ **What are the characteristics of fibromuscular dysplasia in the carotid artery?**

Alternating short intervals of dilatation and stenotic fibromuscular thickenings, turbulence with thromboembolic events, transient ischemic attacks, stroke and intracranial aneurysms.

❏❏ **What are the four types of VSD?**

Perimembranous, supracristal, atrioventricular canal and muscular.

❏❏ **PDA accounts for what percentage of congenital heart defects?**

15%.

❏❏ **What are the boundaries for classification and management of penetrating neck injuries?**

Zone I extends from the clavicle to the cricoid cartilage, zone II extends from the cricoid cartilage to the angle of the mandible and zone III extends from the angle of the mandible to the base of the skull.

❏❏ **Which thoracic surgeries may require one lung ventilation (OLV)?**

Those that involve collapse, retraction or removal of the contralateral lung.

❏❏ **T/F: Mediastenoscopy requires OLV.**

False.

❏❏ **What complications may occur with a double lumen endotracheal tube (DLT)?**

Malpositioning or injury to the trachea or bronchus.

❏❏ **How does CPAP work?**

It maintains the patency of nonventilated alveoli, allowing some oxygen uptake in them.

❏❏ **PDA arises from which aortic arch?**

The left sixth arch.

❏❏ **What is the hallmark of PDA?**

A continuous machinery murmur associated with a widened pulse pressure.

❏❏ **What chest x-ray findings are associated with PDA?**

Left ventricular hypertrophy (LVH), increased vascular markings and an enlarged pulmonary conus.

❏❏ **What is the definitive diagnostic test for PDA?**

Aortography.

❏❏ **What is the treatment of choice for premature infants with PDA?**

Indomethacin.

❏❏ **How much of a shunt is created when OLV is instituted in a healthy lung?**

Approximately 25 to 30%.

❏❏ **What are the indications for bronchoscopy?**

Massive hemoptysis, vascular tumors, endobronchial resection and removal of foreign bodies.

❏❏ **What nerve is most commonly injured during thoracic surgery?**

The intercostal nerve. Branches of the brachial plexus, recurrent laryngeal nerve and the phrenic nerve may also be injured.

❏❏ **What is the anatomy of a bovine aortic arch?**

It is found in approximately 10% of patients undergoing cerebral angiography. The innominate and left common carotid arteries have a common origin.

❏❏ **A 24 year old male with a gunshot wound to the right chest is hemodynamically unstable. The entrance wound is in the second intercostal space, 1 cm lateral to the sternal border. Aortography reveals an injury of the distal innominate artery. What is the most appropriate surgical approach?**

A median sternotomy with supraclavicular extension.

❏❏ **What clinical symptoms are most typical of vertebrobasilar ischemia?**

Diplopia, dizziness, syncope, dysarthria, ataxia and bilateral extremity sensory change and weakness.

❏❏ **What are the diagnostic signs of Takayasu's disease?**

Hypertension, bruits and asymmetric arm pressures.

❏❏ **What is Paget-Schroetter syndrome?**

A syndrome of primary or effort-related thrombosis of the axillary or subclavian vein, caused by compression of the vein during abduction of the arm. Clinical features are those of upper extremity venous hypertension.

❏❏ **What is the subclavian steal syndrome?**

Occlusion of the subclavian artery with subsequent reversed arterial flow from the ipsilateral vertebral artery to the subclavian artery distal to the occlusion.

❏❏ **What is the drainage of the thoracic duct?**

Anatomic variability exists but the thoracic duct usually drains into the proximal left internal jugular vein near its origin.

❏❏ **What is the DeBakey system of aortic dissection classification?**

Type 1 involves the ascending aorta, aortic arch and the thoracoabdominal aorta. Type 2 dissections have a false channel limited to the ascending aorta. Type 3 dissections are divided into 3a (beginning distal to the left subclavian artery and terminating above the diaphragm) and 3b (beginning distal to the left subclavian artery and extending into the abdominal aorta).

❏❏ **Transposition of the great vessels accounts for what percentage of neonatal cyanotic heart disease?**

30 to 40%.

❏❏ **What is the mortality rate for infants with uncorrected transposition of the great vessels?**

90%.

❏❏ **What is the most common location for a recurrent carotid stenosis?**

At the previous endarterectomy site.

❏❏ **What congenital heart lesions result in a continuous (systolic and diastolic) murmur?**

PDA, aortopulmonary window and coronary arteriovenous fistula.

❏❏ **The majority of fetal cardiac development is complete by what gestational age?**

8 weeks.

❏❏ **A 6 month old male presents with sweating and irritability while feeding and chest x-ray demonstrates a markedly enlarged cardiac silhouette. Echocardiogram demonstrates a dilated, poorly contractile left ventricle with moderate to severe mitral regurgitation. What is the diagnosis?**

Anomalous origin of the left coronary artery from the pulmonary artery.

❏❏ **What congenital heart lesion is the most common cause of cyanosis presenting in the newborn period?**

Transposition of the great arteries.

❏❏ **What is the etiology of an atriaventricular (AV) canal defect?**

Underdevelopment of the endocardial cushions leaving a large inlet VSD, a large primum atrial septal defect and a common AV valve separating the atria from the ventricles.

❏❏ **What is the most common late complication of the arterial switch procedure?**

Supravalvular pulmonic stenosis.

❏❏ **Where do aneurysms of the right coronary sinus of Valsalva usually rupture?**

Into the right ventricle.

❏❏ **What are the clinical characteristics of Ebstein's anomaly?**

Varying degrees of deformity of the tricuspid valve with associated obstruction to egress of blood from the right ventricle, severe tricuspid regurgitation and an enlarged cardiac silhouette seen on chest x-ray.

VASCULAR SURGERY PEARLS

*I don't want to achieve mortality through my work.
I want to achieve it through not dying.*
Woody Allen

❏❏ **What type of aortic aneurysm is readily accessible for surgical excision?**

Type C1.

❏❏ **What is stump (back) pressure as used in carotid endarterectomy (CEA)?**

It is thought to reflect the pressure within the Circle of Willis on the operative side of the brain.

❏❏ **What is the minimal accepted value of stump pressure?**

It varies but may be as low as 25 mm Hg.

❏❏ **What does the activated clotting time (ACT) measure?**

Whole blood clotting time; it is also used to evaluate heparinization.

❏❏ **What are the principal cellular elements of the normal vasculature?**

Endothelial cells and smooth muscle cells.

❏❏ **T/F: Back pain is the most common presentation of abdominal aortic aneurysms (AAA).**

False.

❏❏ **What is the etiology of the subclavian steal syndrome?**

Occlusion of the subclavian artery with decreased systolic pressure distal to the obstruction

❏❏ **What is the mechanism of action of heparin?**

Heparin interacts with antithrombin III, a serum protein, resulting in a conformational change in the protein. Antithrombin III then inactivates serine proteases in the coagulation system (XIa, IXa, Xa and IIa). At low doses, the intrinsic pathway is affected, resulting in elevation of the partial thromboplastin time (PTT). At higher doses, the final common pathway is affected, resulting in prolongation of the prothrombin time (PT) as well as the PTT.

❏❏ **T/F: Traumatic thoracic aortic aneurysms are false aneurysms.**

True.

❏❏ **What complications are associated with intraarterial catheters?**

Thrombosis, embolism, pseudoaneurysm, vasospasm, hematoma, infection and arteriovenous fistulae. Median and radial nerve injuries may occur secondary to compression by a hematoma.

❏❏ **What are the signs and symptoms of carotid artery disease (CAD)?**

Transient ischemic attacks (TIAs), reversible ischemic neurologic deficits (RINDs), cerbrovascular accidents (CVAs), amaurosis fugax and bruits.

☐☐ **What are the major determinants of cerebral blood flow (CBF)?**

Arterial CO2 and O2, systemic arterial pressure and temperature.

☐☐ **What factors result in an intraoperative increase in central venous pressure (CVP)?**

Hypervolemia, positive pressure ventilation, Trendelenberg positioning, right ventricular failure, biventricular failure, tricuspid valvular disease, pulmonary hypertension and emboli.

☐☐ **T/F: 50% of patients with cerebral ischemia have a surgically accessible lesion.**

False.

☐☐ **What are the immediate postoperative concerns following CEA?**

CVA, intracerebral hemorrhage, hypertension, hypotension, hematoma, airway obstruction, injury to the recurrent laryngeal, superior laryngeal, hypoglossal or submandibular nerve and vascular headaches.

☐☐ **What is the success rate for percutaneous transluminal angioplasty (PTA) of the iliac arteries?**

95%.

☐☐ **A 76 year old male with a history of hypertension, adult onset diabetes mellitus (DM) and stable angina is undergoing suprarenal aortic aneurysm repair. What type of cardiac evaluation would you recommend preoperatively?**

ECG, electrolytes, chemistry panel, urinalysis, coagulation profile, blood type and screen, noninvasive cardiac testing and angiography.

☐☐ **T/F: Ligation of the inferior mesenteric artery (IMA) can be accomplished with impunity.**

True.

☐☐ **What is the most common complication following AAA repair in a 60 year old male?**

Impotence.

☐☐ **What is the primary effect of lumbar sympathectomy?**

Increased cutaneous circulation.

☐☐ **What are the functions of the venous system?**

Return of blood to the heart from the capillary beds, vascular regulation and thermoregulation.

☐☐ **What conditions are associated with migratory thrombophlebitis?**

Buerger's disease, polyarteritis nodosa and carcinoma of the pancreas.

☐☐ **What is phlegmasia cerulea dolens?**

A deeply cyanotic, painful and massively edematous limb. Most of the deep and superficial venous systems are obstructed with thrombus, restricting venous outflow and, eventually, arterial inflow, leading to venous gangrene.

❏❏ **What are the causes of lower extremity venous hypertension?**

Valvular incompetence, calf pump failure and venous outflow obstruction.

❏❏ **What is the screening test of choice for carotid stenosis?**

Duplex scanning.

❏❏ **What is the most common etiology of advanced venous insufficiency?**

Venous valvular incompetence.

❏❏ **What are the common clinical symptoms of acute pulmonary embolism (PE)?**

Dyspnea, pleural pain, apprehension and cough.

❏❏ **What ECG changes are associated with acute PE?**

Nonspecific ST and T wave changes, wide and deep S waves in lead I, Q waves in lead III and depression of ST-T segments in lead III.

❏❏ **What are the typical arterial blood gas (ABG) changes associated with acute PE?**

Hypoxemia and hypocarbia.

❏❏ **What are the characteristic symptoms of Lariche syndrome?**

Bilateral lower extremity weakness, symmetrical atrophy, pallor of the legs and feet and inability to maintain an erection.

❏❏ **T/F: Intravenous pyelography (IVP) is the diagnostic test of choice for renovascular hypertension.**

False.

❏❏ **What complications are associated with heparin administration?**

Bleeding, heparin-induced thrombocytopenia and hypersensitivity reactions. Chronic heparin use is associated with osteoporosis, alopecia and hypoadrenalism.

❏❏ **What is the result of injury to the hypoglossal nerve?**

Ipsilateral deviation of the tongue and impaired speech and mastication.

❏❏ **What are the indications for axillofemoral bypass?**

An infected aortic aneurysm, infected aortic prosthetic graft and patients who are at excessive risk for abdominal bypass procedures.

❏❏ **What is the most common origin of dissecting aneurysms?**

The ascending aorta.

❏❏ **What is the mechanism of action of Coumadin?**

It inhibits the vitamin K-dependent coagulation factors (II, VII, IX and X).

❏❏ **What are the major side effects of Coumadin?**

Bleeding, skin necrosis and neural tube birth defects.

❏❏ **What are the complications of iliofemoral venous thrombectomy?**

PE, early re-thrombosis and wound complications.

❏❏ **What is a papaverine test?**

When injected directly into a peripheral artery, papaverine causes a temporary increase in flow to the limb. The presence of significant stenosis proximal to the injection point will cause a sudden, temporary decrease in the intraarterial pressure measured below that point.

❏❏ **What are the major indications for infrarenal vena cava (Greenfield) filter placement?**

Documented lower extremity deep vein thrombosis (DVT) or PE with a recognized contraindication to anticoagulation, PE despite adequate anticoagulation, bleeding complications of anticoagulation and after pulmonary embolectomy.

❏❏ **What are the most common complications of prosthetic arterial grafts?**

Fibrous hyperplasia, infection, graft failure and formation of false aneurysms.

❏❏ **What is the most important factor contributing to flow through a stenotic artery?**

The diameter of the stenosis.

❏❏ **What complications are associated with the use of a Greenfield filter?**

Failure of insertion, incomplete opening, leg asymmetry, perforation of the inferior vena cava (IVC), hematoma at the insertion site, filter movement, recurrent PE and caval thrombosis.

❏❏ **What is the most common site of occlusion in cardioarterial emboli?**

The common femoral artery.

❏❏ **What factors contribute to the development of primary varicose veins?**

Valvular incompetence, weakness of the vein wall and presence of multiple arteriovenous fistulae.

❏❏ **What is the most common site of origin of traumatic thoracic aorta aneurysms?**

Just distal to the origin of the left subclavian vein.

❏❏ **What are the indications for surgical treatment of varicose veins?**

Leg pain, edema, episodes of recurrent thrombophlebitis and cosmesis.

❏❏ **Which veins are ideally treated with sclerotherapy?**

Cosmetically unsightly telangiectasias, reticular varicosities and small isolated varicosities in the absence of saphenofemoral reflux.

❏❏ **How do sclerosing agents work?**

By inducing thrombosis and fibrosis.

❏❏ **What are the main complications from the use of sclerosants?**

Anaphylactic reactions, epidermal necrosis, hyperpigmentation, blistering and ulceration.

❏❏ What is the cause of skin ulceration in a patient with chronic venous insufficiency?

White blood cell trapping within the skin microcirculation, leading to microvascular congestion and thrombosis. The WBCs migrate into the interstitium and release lysosomal enzymes, resulting in tissue destruction.

❏❏ What is May Turner Syndrome?

Compression of the left iliac vein by the right common iliac artery.

❏❏ What are the criteria for diagnosis of lower extremity claudication?

Leg pain with exertion, relieved by rest and elevation, ipsilateral iliac vein obstruction, venous hypertension at rest and elevation of venous pressure with exercise.

❏❏ What are the propulsive forces for lymphatic flow?

Spontaneous, intrinsic, segmental muscular contractions, breathing, sighing, yawning, muscular squeezing and transmitted arterial pulsations.

❏❏ What is the most common causative organism of cellulitis in a lymphedematous limb?

Beta-hemolytic streptococcus.

❏❏ What is the most common vasospastic disorder affecting women less than 40 years of age?

Raynaud's disease/phenomenon.

❏❏ What are the etiologic classifications of lymphedema?

Primary lymphedema may be congenital, praecox or tarda. Secondary lymphedema may result from surgical removal of the lymphatics, infection or malignancy.

❏❏ What is the most frequent cause of secondary lymphedema in North America and Europe?

Surgical excision and irradiation of the axillary or inguinal lymph nodes for malignancy.

❏❏ What are the early skin manifestations of lymphedema?

The skin has a pinkish-red color and a mildly elevated temperature.

❏❏ What are the complications of contrast lymphangiography?

Obstructive lymphangitis, progression of lymphedema, pulmonary embolization of oily contrast material and allergic reactions.

❏❏ What is the proper method for determination of the ankle-brachial index (ABI)?

A standard brachial blood pressure cuff is placed around the ankle, just above the malleoli. A hand-held Doppler is used to measure the pressures in the dorsalis pedis and posterior tibial arteries. Both brachial blood pressures are determined, also using the Doppler. The ABI is calculated by dividing the highest ankle pressure by the highest brachial pressure.

❏❏ What is the relationship between the finding of a carotid bruit on physical examination and the degree of carotid stenosis?

Almost none.

❏❏ **What is the typical early presentation of a patient with acute mesenteric ischemia?**

Severe, generalized abdominal pain with a remarkably benign abdominal examination. There may also be nausea, vomiting or diarrhea.

❏❏ **What is phlegmasia alba dolens?**

A painful, swollen, white leg that results from an iliofemoral DVT and resulting in extremity edema.

❏❏ **What is the post-phlebitic syndrome?**

A constellation of signs and symptoms that relate to lower extremity venous insufficiency. The patient usually has chronic lower extremity edema, a brownish discoloration of the skin and ulcerations in the medial malleolar region.

❏❏ **What is the typical presentation of a patient with chronic mesenteric ischemia?.**

Intermittent post-prandial epigastric pain that begins 30 to 60 minutes after eating and may persist for a few hours.

❏❏ **What are 6 P's of acute arterial occlusion?**

Pain, pallor, pulselessness, paresthesias, paralysis and poikilothermia.

❏❏ **T/F: The absence of a Doppler signal indicates the absence of flow.**

False.

❏❏ **What diseases are associated with occlusive tibioperoneal atherosclerosis?**

Diabetes mellitus and Buerger's disease.

❏❏ **Considering duplex testing, what are the broad categories of carotid arterial stenosis?**

Normal, 0 to 15%, 16 to 49%, 50 to 79%, 80 to 99% and total occlusion.

❏❏ **What are the most common complications of arteriography?**

Renal failure, allergic reaction to contrast media, hematoma, pseudoaneurysm and arteriovenous fistulae.

❏❏ **Repair of which type of aneurysm is associated with the highest operative mortality rate?**

Transverse aortic arch aneurysms.

❏❏ **What medications are used in thrombolysis and what is their mechanism of action?**

Streptokinase forms an activated complex with plasminogen. This complex converts excess plasminogen to plasmin. Urokinase acts directly on plasminogen to form plasmin. Tissue plasminogen activator (tPA) directly activates plasminogen already bound to a fibrin clot.

❏❏ **What cardiovascular risk factors most influence the perioperative outcome for patients with vascular disease undergoing noncardiac surgery?**

Myocardial infarction (MI) within 6 months, worsening or unstable angina pectoris, symptomatic aortic valvular stenosis, symptomatic congestive heart failure (CHF), chronic atrial or ventricular dysrhythmias, chronic obstructive pulmonary disease (COPD), chronic renal insufficiency, hepatic insufficiency and malnutrition.

❏❏ **What nerves are at risk during carotid surgery?**

The hypoglossal, vagus, superior laryngeal, greater auricular and the mandibular branch of the facial nerve.

❏❏ **What common conditions mimic claudication?**

Sciatic nerve root disorders, arthritis, chronic venous insufficiency, proximal venous obstruction, diabetic neuropathy and marked obesity.

❏❏ **What is the diagnostic test of choice for AAA?**

Computed tomography for initial non-emergent diagnosis. Ultrasonography is most useful for following progression of aneurysmal dilatation.

❏❏ **T/F: Slow rewarming is the treatment of choice for frostbite.**

False.

❏❏ **What is the natural history of claudication?**

Fewer than 10% of patients with claudication will progress to critical ischemia or amputation. Most of those who do progress have uncontrolled risk factors, diabetes mellitus or continue to smoke.

❏❏ **What are the characteristic chest x-ray findings of aortic injury?**

Widening of the mediastinum, blunting of the aortic knob, left apical capping, deviation of the trachea to the right and depression of the left mainstem bronchus.

❏❏ **What are the medical and behavioral treatments for claudication?**

Management of risk factors is essential (i.e., cessation of smoking and control of diabetes, hyperlipidemia and blood pressure are the initial maneuvers). A supervised time-based walking exercise program, especially in the absence of smoking, will build collaterals, lessen symptoms and increase walking tolerance. Trental may increase the walking distance in some claudicants.

❏❏ **What are the requirements for successful arterial reconstruction?**

Adequate inflow, adequate outflow and an adequate conduit.

❏❏ **What is the tri-modal distribution of graft failure?**

Technical error, intimal hyperplasia and progression of atherosclerotic disease.

❏❏ **How does the location of the distal anastomosis relate to graft patency?**

In general, the more distal the anastomosis, the lower the graft patency.

❏❏ **What is a pseudoaneurysm?**

An enlargement of a vascular circuit lacking the full layers of the vessel wall.

❏❏ **What are the common clinical presentations of chronic lower extremity ischemia?**

Ischemic rest pain, chronic skin ulceration and gangrene.

❏❏ **What factors are predictive of healing following amputation?**

A segmental arterial pressure of 50 mm Hg at the level of the planned amputation and a TcPO2 greater than 50 Torr for the skin flap.

❏❏ **What are the most common technical problems following an in situ bypass?**

A missed valve cusp and a missed vein branch.

❏❏ **What is the role of debridement in diabetic foot infections?**

Extensive debridement and wide exposure of all devitalized tissue and underlying bone.

❏❏ **How does amputation change the work of walking?**

A unilateral below-knee amputation (BKA) increases the work of walking by 50%, 100% for unilateral above-knee amputations (AKAs).

❏❏ **What is the natural history of AAAs?**

They expand in diameter with gradually increasing wall tension until the burst strength is exceeded.

❏❏ **What is the difference between saccular and fusiform aneurysms?**

The usual aortic aneurysm is fusiform, where the dilation involves the entire circumference of the vessel. Many visceral and cerebral aneurysms are saccular, where the majority of the vessel circumference may be normal in caliber with only a portion of the circumference weakening and dilating.

❏❏ **What is the natural history of popliteal artery aneurysms?**

It tends to thrombose acutely and cause limb-threatening ischemia.

❏❏ **What is the relationship of a popliteal aneurysm to an AAA?**

Approximately 20% of patients with an AAA have a popliteal aneurysm. 40 to 60% of patients with a unilateral popliteal aneurysm have an AAA.

❏❏ **What is the mechanism of renovascular hypertension?**

The renal juxtaglomerular apparatus (JGA), through the renin-angiotensin system, seeks to maintain a normal arterial pressure at the JGA. Stenotic arterial lesions proximal to the kidney cause the JGA to secrete renin, which through the angiotensin cascade, raises the central pressure above normal and, therefore, the pressure at the JGA (beyond the stenosis) rises towards normal.

❏❏ **What is the thoracic outlet?**

An anatomic region formed by the first rib, clavicle and scalene muscles through which pass the brachial plexus, subclavian artery and subclavian vein. The nerves and artery are posterior to the vein and separated by the anterior scalene muscle.

❏❏ **What is thoracic outlet syndrome?**

Anything that narrows the outlet, such as muscular hypertrophy, fibrous tissue, cervical ribs, scar tissue or fracture callus, can impinge on one or more of the structures within it.

❏❏ **What is Virchow's Triad?**

Stasis, endothelial cell injury and a hypercoagulable state.

❑❑ **What patients are at increased risk for DVT?**

Those with hypercoagulable body chemistries, previous DVT, lower-extremity trauma, orthopedic surgery, major pelvic operations, immobility, acute MI, CHF, malignancies and those taking oral contraceptives, especially if they smoke.

❑❑ **What are the effective prophylactic measures for DVT?**

Coumadin, unfractionated heparin, low-molecular weight heparins, dextran, antiplatelet drugs such as aspirin or ticlid and sequential venous compression stockings (SCDs).

CHEST WALL, LUNG, PLEURA AND MEDIASTINUM PEARLS

The best way to stop smoking is to carry wet matches.
Anonymous

❑❑ T/F: Total lung capacity (TLC) is equal to the functional residual capacity (FRC) plus the vital capacity (VC).

False.

❑❑ When performing a posterolateral thoracotomy, what chest wall muscles are usually transected?

The latissimus dorsi and serratus anterior.

❑❑ The inferior pulmonary vein of the lung lies within what structure?

The pulmonary ligament.

❑❑ Through what anatomic structure are the pulmonary artery branches approached during lower lobectomy?

The major fissure.

❑❑ Why is the most common site of aspiration pneumonia the lower lobe of the right lung?

Aspirated contents and foreign bodies are more likely to go to the right since the right mainstem bronchus is shorter, more vertical and wider than the left mainstem bronchus. The lower lobe orifices lie more posterior and are the more likely site of aspiration, especially when supine.

❑❑ Horner's syndrome is most often associated with which intrathoracic malignancy?

A superior sulcus (Pancoast) tumor.

❑❑ T/F: At the level of the carina, the pulmonary arteries lie anterior to the mainstem bronchus and posterior to the aortic arch.

True.

❑❑ What is the most common form of non-small cell lung cancer in the United States?

Adenocarcinoma.

❑❑ T/F: Paraneoplastic syndromes occur most commonly in small cell lung cancer.

True.

❑❑ T/F: Small cell lung cancer is often widely disseminated at the time of diagnosis and is infrequently treated with surgical resection.

True.

☐☐ T/F: Solitary pulmonary nodules found in patients over 50 years old are more likely to contain malignancy than those found in younger patients.

True.

☐☐ Following a history, physical examination and chest x-rays, what constitutes the minimum preoperative evaluation for staging of patients with non-small cell lung cancer?

Complete blood count, liver function tests, serum electrolytes, computed tomography of the chest and upper abdomen and bronchoscopy.

☐☐ What are the common sites for metastases from lung cancer?

The brain, adrenal glands, bone, liver, contralateral lung and mediastinal and supraclavicular lymph nodes.

☐☐ What is the most common benign tumor of the lung?

Hamartoma.

☐☐ Which type of non small cell lung cancer is often multicentric, metastasizes via aerosolization within the lung and requires extended follow-up?

Bronchoalveolar carcinoma.

☐☐ Which lung neoplasm in young to middle-aged patients is often centrally located, usually endobronchial and may present with obstructive symptoms or hemoptysis?

Bronchopulmonary carcinoid.

☐☐ What criteria must be met for a patient to benefit from resection of metastases to the lung?

The primary tumor must be controlled or controllable, metastatic disease confined to the lung and complete resection with adequate residual pulmonary function.

☐☐ What is the preferred technique for the resection of metastases to the lung?

Wedge resection.

☐☐ T/F: The resection of metastases to the lung increases the overall median survival in selected patients.

True.

☐☐ What is the most common postoperative complication following pulmonary resection?

Atelectasis.

☐☐ What is the most likely cause of severe head, neck and arm swelling in a patient with a centrally located mass on chest x-ray?

The superior vena cava syndrome.

☐☐ What is the standard therapy for a lung abscess?

Systemic antibiotics and bronchoscopy to remove any foreign body and to exclude endobronchial tumor or obstruction.

❏❏ Which type of alveolar lining epithelial cell produces surfactant?

Type II pneumocytes.

❏❏ Which microaerophillic bacterium can produce lung abscesses and sinus tracts that drain yellow-brown material resembling sulfur granules?

Actinomycosis.

❏❏ What is the most common cause of massive hemoptysis (greater than 600 ml of blood in 24 hours)?

Tuberculosis.

❏❏ What term is used to describe the over expansion of a pulmonary lobe that can be a cause of respiratory distress in infants?

Lobar emphysema.

❏❏ T/F: A 60 year old patient with a preoperative FEV1 of 1.8 and a ventilation-perfusion (V/Q) scan showing 60% function from the left lung is not at increased risk of postoperative respiratory insufficiency following left pneumonectomy.

True.

❏❏ What form of bronchopulmonary sequestration shares a common pleural investment with the normal pulmonary tissue, derives its blood supply from a large systemic artery and may communicate with the tracheobronchial tree?

Intralobar sequestration.

❏❏ Blunt trauma to the chest, pneumomediastinum, subcutaneous emphysema and a large air leak following tube thoracostomy all imply what type of injury?

A tracheobronchial tear or disruption.

❏❏ What is the definitive method of diagnosing a tracheobronchial injury?

Bronchoscopy.

❏❏ The sudden onset of a continuous cough with copious serosanguinous or purulent sputum while a patient is recovering from pneumonectomy is pathognomonic for what condition?

A postoperative bronchopleural fistula.

❏❏ What are the risk factors for postoperative bronchopleural fistula following pulmonary resection?

Diabetes mellitus, malnutrition, radiation therapy, infection, inflammation or devascularization of the bronchial stump and residual tumor at the site of bronchial closure.

❏❏ What protozoon is responsible for a diffuse interstitial pneumonitis in immunocompromised patients?

Pneumocystis carinii.

❏❏ T/F: Pre-thoracotomy diagnosis of ipsilateral mediastinal lymph node metastases from non-small cell lung cancer precludes curative resection of the primary tumor.

True.

❏❏ **T/F: Patients with pulmonary arteriovenous malformations should undergo resection or embolization because of their associated complications.**

True.

❏❏ **What are the possible complications of mediastinoscopy?**

Bleeding, injury to the left recurrent laryngeal nerve, esophageal perforation, pneumothorax and infection.

❏❏ **What is the clinical significance of ipsilateral supraclavicular lymph node metastases from non-small cell lung cancer?**

These are considered N3 nodal metastases and preclude curative resection of the primary lung tumor.

❏❏ **What are the anatomic boundaries of the mediastinum?**

Superior – thoracic inlet
Inferior – diaphragm
Anterior – sternum
Posterior – vertebral bodies
Lateral – mediastinal pleura

❏❏ **What is acute descending necrotizing mediastinitis?**

A necrotizing inflammatory process resulting from extension of an oropharyngeal infection. It is often accompanied by empyema and/or acute pericarditis.

❏❏ **When postoperative infection is excluded, what is responsible for approximately 90% of cases of acute mediastinitis?**

Esophageal perforation.

❏❏ **How does a pneumothorax result in collapse of the lung parenchyma?**

Intrapleural pressure rises above intrabronchial pressure.

❏❏ **How does a large pneumothorax produce arterial hypoxemia?**

By producing a shunt.

❏❏ **What is the etiology of Hamman's sign?**

Pneumomediastinum.

❏❏ **What is the best way to distinguish a pneumothorax from large lung bullae?**

CT scan.

❏❏ **What is the most common cause of a spontaneous pneumothorax?**

Rupture of a pulmonary bleb.

❏❏ **What are the recurrence rates for an ipsilateral spontaneous pneumothorax following a first, second or third episode?**

30, 50 and 80%, respectively.

❏❏ **What are the most common primary malignant tumors of the chest wall?**

Myeloma and chondrosarcoma.

❏❏ **What is the most common benign tumor of the chest wall?**

An osteochondroma.

❏❏ **What is the most common indication for pectus carinatum repair?**

Cosmetic improvement.

❏❏ **What is the most common underlying lung disease in elderly patients who are diagnosed with a spontaneous pneumothorax?**

Chronic obstructive pulmonary disease.

❏❏ **What are the indications for surgical treatment of a spontaneous pneumothorax?**

Massive air leak preventing lung re-expansion, air leak persisting longer than 5 to 7 days, ipsilateral recurrence, simultaneous bilateral pneumothoraces, presentation with tension pneumothorax, associated empyema or hemothorax and lifestyle indications (i.e., airline pilot, scuba diver and resides in remote area).

❏❏ **What technique should be combined with bleb resection in the surgical treatment of a pneumothorax?**

Mechanical pleurodesis or pleurectomy.

❏❏ **What potential advantages might thoracoscopic surgery have over conventional surgical techniques in treating spontaneous pneumothoraces?**

Easier examination of all lung surfaces, less postoperative pain, shorter hospital stay and earlier return to work.

❏❏ **What are the complications of a prolonged chylothorax?**

Protein malnutrition, intravascular volume loss and decreased cellular immunity secondary to the loss of circulating T cells.

❏❏ **What is the initial management of a patient with a chylothorax?**

Thoracostomy tube drainage, maintenance of fluid and electrolytes, bowel rest and parenteral nutrition.

❏❏ **What type of chest x-ray is helpful in distinguishing a pleural effusion from other intrathoracic densities?**

A lateral decubitus.

❏❏ **What is the generally accepted etiology of pectus excavatum?**

Misdirected rapid growth of the lower costal cartilages in a concave manner, creating a depressed sternum.

❏❏ **When trauma and pulmonary infarction are excluded, what is responsible for 90% of bloody pleural effusions?**

Malignancy.

❏❏ **What laboratory values suggest that a pleural effusion is an exudate?**

A pleural fluid/serum protein ratio greater than 0.5 and a pleural fluid/serum LDH ratio greater than 0.6.

❑❑ **What causes of persistent pleural effusions are readily diagnosed by pleural biopsy?**

Tuberculosis and malignancy involving the pleura.

❑❑ **What is considered an adequate margin of resecting for a primary chest wall malignancy?**

4 cm circumferential margins of the chest wall including any involved lung, pericardium, diaphragm, chest wall muscles or skin.

❑❑ **What are the goals of decortication in the setting of a hemothorax refractory to tube thoracostomy drainage?**

Relieve pulmonary entrapment, preserve pulmonary function and prevent empyema formation.

❑❑ **What technique is 90% successful in identifying the etiology of pleural effusions undiagnosed after thoracentesis and pleural biopsy?**

Thoracoscopy.

❑❑ **What is the most common origin of an anterior mediastinal mass in an adult?**

The thymus.

❑❑ **What is the most common posterior mediastinal tumor?**

A neurogenic tumor.

❑❑ **What diagnostic study is most useful for defining a mediastinal mass identified on chest x-ray?**

CT scan of the chest with oral and intravenous contrast.

❑❑ **What serum studies should be obtained in male patients with a mediastinal mass?**

Alpha-fetoprotein (AFP) and human chorionic gonadotropin (HCG).

❑❑ **What is the most common mediastinal tumor in children less than 2 years old?**

A neurogenic tumor.

❑❑ **Why should asymptomatic mediastinal tumors of neurogenic origin be resected?**

To provide histologic confirmation if it's benign nature, prevent the local effects of progressive enlargement and to prevent malignant degeneration.

❑❑ **What percentage of patients with a thymoma have myasthenia gravis (MG)?**

50%.

❑❑ **T/F: A solitary pulmonary nodule that has not changed in appearance on chest x-ray over 6 months is likely to be benign and can be followed with yearly radiographs.**

False.

❑❑ **What percentage of thymic masses are malignant?**

33%.

☐☐ **What is the most common mediastinal tumor in adults?**

A neurogenic tumor.

☐☐ **What incision provides the best exposure for resecting a mass located in the anterior mediastinum?**

A median sternotomy.

☐☐ **What is the most common cause of a large pleural effusion?**

Malignancy.

☐☐ **What percentage of patients with MG will show clinical improvement following resection of a thymoma?**

85 to 95%.

☐☐ **T/F: Posterior mediastinal masses in adults are most often malignant.**

False.

☐☐ **What treatment is required for a bronchogenic cyst?**

Surgical excision to alleviate symptoms, establish a histologic diagnosis and prevent possible malignant degeneration.

☐☐ **T/F: Pericardial cysts often occur in the right pericardiophrenic angle, can usually be diagnosed by CT scan and infrequently require surgical excision.**

True.

☐☐ **What is the most common cause of a malignant pleural effusion?**

Carcinoma of the lung.

☐☐ **What are the treatment goals for patients with a pleural empyema?**

Control of local infection with drainage and systemic antibiotics, re-expansion of the lung and obliteration of the pleural space.

☐☐ **What compensatory measures obliterate the intrathoracic space left by pulmonary resection?**

Mediastinal shift, elevation of the ipsilateral hemidiaphragm, contraction of the intercostal spaces and expansion of the remaining ipsilateral pulmonary parenchyma.

☐☐ **What intrathoracic neoplasms are associated with asbestos exposure?**

Malignant mesothelioma and lung cancer.

☐☐ **What is the most common intrathoracic neoplasm among cigarette smokers with a history of asbestos exposure?**

Bronchogenic lung carcinoma.

☐☐ **T/F: Malignant mesothelioma usually presents with chest wall pain and dyspnea and has documented asbestos exposure in only 50% of patients.**

True.

LIVER, GALLBLADDER, PANCREAS AND SPLEEN PEARLS

Confirmed dispepsia is the apparatus of illusions.
George Meredith

❏❏ **What are the most common causes of acute pancreatitis?**

Alcohol and gallstones.

❏❏ **How might a patient with a VIPoma (Werner-Morrison syndrome) (WDHA) present?**

With hypokalemia, achlorhydria and watery diarrhea.

❏❏ **What drugs are known to cause pancreatitis.**

Sulfonamides, estrogens, tetracyclines, pentamidine, azathioprine, thiazides, furosemide and valproic acid.

❏❏ **What are the infectious causes of pancreatitis?**

Mumps, viral hepatitis, Coxsackie virus group B and mycoplasma.

❏❏ **How much hepatic bile is produced daily?**

Approximately 600 ml.

❏❏ **What are the common symptoms of acute pancreatitis?**

Epigastric or diffuse abdominal pain radiating to the back, nausea and vomiting.

❏❏ **T/F: Acute pancreatitis commonly progresses to chronic pancreatitis.**

False.

❏❏ **Why can portal venous pressure be measured at any point in the system?**

Because the portal vein is valveless.

❏❏ **What are the laboratory abnormalities in pancreatitis?**

Leukocytosis, hemoconcentration, anemia, hyperglycemia, prerenal azotemia, hypoxemia, hyperamylasemia and liver function test (LFT) abnormalities.

❏❏ **Why is hyperamylasemia central to the diagnosis of pancreatitis?**

Widespread availability, low cost, it has a sensitivity of 89% and a specificity of 86%.

❏❏ **T/F: Normal amylase levels rule out pancreatitis.**

False. Amylase peaks within a few hours of an attack and then declines.

❏❏ **T/F: The level of amylase elevation correlates with severity of pancreatitis.**

False. Higher levels are seen in biliary pancreatitis.

❏❏ **What findings on abdominal x-ray are consistent with pancreatitis?**

Generalized ileus, sentinel loops, the colon cutoff sign, biliary calcifications and pancreatic calcifications.

❏❏ **What is the role of CT scanning in pancreatitis?**

For diagnosis, to assess severity, detect complications and as a guide to aspiration and drainage of fluid collections.

❏❏ **How is endoscopic retrograde cholangiopancreatography (ERCP) useful in patients with pancreatitis?**

It can establish ductal disruption in traumatic pancreatitis and it may be useful in early cases of acute biliary pancreatitis.

❏❏ **T/F: Hydroxylation of vitamin D by cytochrome P-450 occurs in the liver.**

False.

❏❏ **What is the most appropriate treatment for a patient with a subcapsular hematoma following blunt trauma?**

Observation.

❏❏ **What are the Ranson's criteria for severity in acute nonbiliary pancreatitis on admission?**

Age greater than 55 years, WBC count greater than 16,000/mm3, glucose greater than 200 mg/dl, LDH greater than 350 U/l and AST greater than 250 U/l.

❏❏ **What are the Ranson's criteria for severity of biliary pancreatitis at 48 hours?**

A fall in hematocrit of greater than 10%, a rise in BUN greater than 2%, calcium less than 8 mg/dl, base deficit greater than 5 mEq/l and fluid sequestration greater than 4 liters.

❏❏ **What is the simplified Glasgow prognostic criteria in pancreatitis?**

Age greater than 55 years, WBC count greater than 15,000/mm3, glucose greater than 180 mg/dl, LDH greater than 600 U/l, BUN greater than 45 mg/dl, calcium less than 8 mg/dl, albumin less than 32 gm/l and $PaCO_2$ less than 60 mm Hg.

❏❏ **T/F: Cholecystokinin inhibits bile flow.**

True.

❏❏ **What is the preferred analgesic for pancreatitis?**

Meperidine.

❏❏ **What is the initial treatment for patients with pancreatitis?**

NPO until near complete resolution of pain and tenderness.

❏❏ **What are the septic complications of pancreatitis?**

Pancreatic abscess, infected pseudocyst and infected fluid collections.

❏❏ **T/F: Leucine aminopeptidase is elevated in patients with obstructive jaundice.**

False.

❏❏ **What is the diagnostic test of choice for the complications of pancreatitis?**

CT scan.

❏❏ **When is surgery indicated for patients with complications of pancreatitis?**

In cases of infected pancreatic necrosis and for abscesses that cannot be adequately drained percutaneously.

❏❏ **T/F: Immediate surgery should be performed in patients with gallstone pancreatitis.**

False.

❏❏ **What is the nature of the pleural fluid in pancreatitis?**

It is an exudate with high amylase levels.

❏❏ **T/F: Pleuropulmonary complications indicate severe disease in patients with pancreatitis.**

True.

❏❏ **What is the mortality rate for patients with pancreatitis who require mechanical ventilation?**

75%.

❏❏ **What is the differential diagnosis of acute pancreatitis?**

Cholecystitis, perforated viscus, penetrating ulcer, hepatitis, intestinal obstruction, mesenteric ischemia, vasculitis, myocardial infarction (MI), pneumonia, renal colic, diabetic ketoacidosis (DKA) and appendicitis.

❏❏ **What is a pancreatic pseudocyst?**

A collection of necrotic tissue with fluid and blood that develops near the pancreas over a period of 1 to 4 weeks. Pseudocysts do not have a true capsule.

❏❏ **What are the complications of pancreatic pseudocysts?**

Infection, perforation and hemorrhage.

❏❏ **What are the clinical features of chronic pancreatitis?**

Abdominal pain, pancreatic calcifications, malabsorption and diabetes mellitus (DM).

❏❏ **What is the etiology of chronic pancreatitis?**

Progressive damage and permanent destruction of exocrine and endocrine functions.

❏❏ **What is the appropriate treatment for a patient with a type I choledochal cyst?**

Cyst excision.

❏❏ **What is the blood supply to the liver?**

75% is derived from the portal vein and 25% from the hepatic artery. The hepatic oxygen supply, however, is derived equally from the hepatic arteries and the portal vein.

❑❑ **How does anesthesia affect liver blood flow?**

Regional anesthesia has minimal effects on liver blood flow unless it is accompanied by hypotension. General anesthesia uniformly decreases liver blood flow by approximately 20 to 30%.

❑❑ **T/F: Esophageal varices bleed by erosion.**

False.

❑❑ **What acid-base abnormalities are seen in patients with cirrhosis?**

Mild to moderate hypoxemia and respiratory alkalosis.

❑❑ **What are the sites of arteriovenous shunts in patients with chronic liver disease?**

Skin (spider nevi), muscles, intrahepatic and intrapulmonary.

❑❑ **What percentage of patients with gallstones are candidates for dissolution therapy?**

15%.

❑❑ **What are the indications for gallstone dissolution therapy?**

Stones that are less than 5 mm and noncalcified and a gallbladder that opacifies on an oral cholecystogram (indicating patency of the cystic duct). Dissolution therapy, commonly with ursodiol, is effective in dissolving 50% of stones within 2 years.

❑❑ **What patient populations are at risk for acute acalculous cholecystitis?**

Trauma patients and those requiring long-term TPN.

❑❑ **What electrolyte abnormalities are seen in patients with chronic liver disease?**

Hyponatremia, hypophosphatemia and hypocalcemia.

❑❑ **Why are patients with fulminant hepatic failure (FHF) prone to hypoglycemia?**

Secondary to depletion of glycogen stores in the liver and decreased glycogenolysis and glucose regulating hormone interactions.

❑❑ **T/F: Patients with cirrhosis are prone to hypoglycemia.**

True.

❑❑ **What are the vitamin K dependent coagulation factors?**

Factors II, VII, IX, X, protein C and protein S.

❑❑ **A patient with massive ascites is scheduled for peritoneovenous (LeVeen) shunt placement. How would you secure the airway?**

By rapid sequence induction.

❑❑ **What is the primary long-term complication of bile duct injuries?**

Bile duct stricture.

❑❑ **T/F: Placement of an intracranial pressure (ICP) monitor is contraindicated in patients with fulminant hepatic failure.**

True.

❑❑ **T/F: Patients with obstructive jaundice are prone to renal failure.**

True.

❑❑ **What are the hemodynamic consequence of inferior vena cava (IVC) cross clamping?**

It decreases venous return by as much as 45%, resulting in decreased cardiac output and hypotension.

❑❑ **What are the main postoperative complications following orthotopic liver transplantation (OLT)?**

Rejection and infection.

❑❑ **What plane separates the right lobe of the liver from the left lobe?**

The plane is defined by the gallbladder bed, the retrohepatic vena cava and the junction of the right and middle hepatic veins.

❑❑ **What is the most common cause of choledochoduodenal fistulas?**

Penetrating peptic ulcers.

❑❑ **What vein enters the retrohepatic vena cava (other than the hepatic veins)?**

The right adrenal vein.

❑❑ **Where are primary bile salts converted to secondary bile salts?**

In the small intestine and colon.

❑❑ **What are the complications of total portosystemic shunts?**

Encephalopathy and hepatic failure.

❑❑ **What is the origin of the blood supply to the bile duct?**

It arises superiorly from the hepatic artery and inferiorly from the pancreaticoduodenal arcades. There are also blood vessels on the lateral edges of the duct.

❑❑ **Unconjugated hyperbilirubinemia, without other liver function abnormality, is most likely due to what disorders?**

Neonatal hyperbilirubinemia, Crigler-Najjar type I and II and Gilbert's disease.

❑❑ **What is delta bilirubin?**

Conjugated bilirubin that is covalently bound to albumin.

❑❑ **What is the significance of delta bilirubin?**

It accumulates in large quantities in patients with chronic conjugated hyperbilirubinemia and persists after the underlying problem is corrected and the bound albumin is metabolized.

❏❏ **What is the role of vitamin K in the synthesis of coagulation factors?**

It is a cofactor in the gamma-carboxylation of factors II, VI, IX and X. These factors are inactive without this carboxylation.

❏❏ **How is the liver involved in the Cori cycle?**

Lactate, produced by anaerobic metabolism in the tissues, is converted to pyruvate almost exclusively in the liver.

❏❏ **How is the endothelial lining of the hepatic sinusoid different from other capillaries, and what is its significance?**

It has large fenestrations. Consequently, it has a permeability of about 30 times that of other capillaries. Thus, filtration through the sinusoid is much faster. In addition, there is a space on the tissue side of the sinusoid (the space of Disse) giving the hepatocyte a large surface for contact with the filtered fluid in the extravascular space.

❏❏ **What is the significance of elevation of the serum transaminases AST (SGOT) and ALT (SGPT)?**

These enzymes are released from hepatocytes when they are injured or die. ALT is more hepatocyte-specific while AST can be elevated with red cell, muscle cell or cardiac muscle cell death. They are not measures of liver cell function.

❏❏ **What is a strawberry gallbladder?**

Deposition of cholesterol in macrophages (foamy histiocytes) within the lamina propria of the gallbladder wall.

❏❏ **What is the most common nodule in the liver?**

An hemangioma.

❏❏ **What complications are associated with acute cholecystitis?**

Perforation, gangrene and empyema.

❏❏ **What are the elements of Charcot's triad?**

Jaundice, fever with chills and biliary colic.

❏❏ **What organisms are most commonly involved in bacterial cholangitis?**

E. coli, klebsiella, pseudomonas, enterococci and proteus.

❏❏ **What are the common complications of choledocholithiasis?**

Secondary biliary cirrhosis, acute pancreatitis and intrahepatic abscesses.

❏❏ **How is the caudate lobe different from the other segments of the liver, with respect to its vascular supply?**

It receives blood from the right and left hepatic arteries and the portal vein. Most of the venous blood drains directly into the vena cava.

❏❏ **What percentage of normal persons have classic hepatic arterial anatomy (a single hepatic artery arising from the celiac axis and dividing into the left and right hepatic arteries)?**

50%.

❏❏ **What therapy is indicated for a patient with an amebic abscess?**

Metronidazole, 400 mg TID for 4 days or a single dose of 2.5 gm combined with aspiration.

❏❏ **What is the most common type of malignant liver carcinoma?**

Hepatocellular.

❏❏ **What are the risk factors for hepatocellular carcinoma (HCC)?**

Aflatoxins, low protein intake, hepatitis B and C and cirrhosis.

❏❏ **How is alpha-fetoprotein (AFP) helpful in following patients with cirrhosis for the development of cancer?**

A rising AFP predicts development of HCC.

❏❏ **What is an adequate margin of resection for hepatocellular cancer?**

1 cm.

❏❏ **How does cirrhosis affect the outcome of liver resection?**

The cirrhotic liver regenerates poorly and may not fully recover after extensive liver resection. Hepatic failure may ensue.

❏❏ **Positive bile cultures are most often associated with what condition?**

Postoperative bile duct stricture.

❏❏ **What are the most common benign hepatic lesions?**

Hepatic adenomas, hemangiomas, focal nodular hyperplasia and hepatic cysts.

❏❏ **What are the most frequently used tests to differentiate these lesions?**

Ultrasound, a technetium sulfur colloid scan and dynamic CT angiogram.

❏❏ **What intraoperative factors can influence the outcome of liver resection in the cirrhotic patient?**

Blood loss, hepatic ischemia and the amount of remaining liver.

❏❏ **What factors influence survival in patients with hepatocellular carcinoma?**

Large tumor size (greater than 5 cm) and patients with satellite lesions have poor survival rates. Vascular invasion, a small margin of resection and portal vein thrombosis are also poor prognostic indicators. Encapsulated and fibrolamellar tumors have better survival.

❏❏ **What palliative treatments are available for the management of unresectable HCC?**

Chemoembolization, injection of alcohol into smaller tumors and cryoablation.

❏❏ **What is the value of PET scanning in the evaluation of patients with colorectal metastases to the liver?**

It may allow identification of additional lesions in the liver or outside the liver, that may render curative resection impossible.

❏❏ **What percentage of patients with colorectal cancer have hepatic metastases when the primary is discovered?**

20%.

❏❏ **T/F: The presence of extrahepatic disease is a contraindication to resection of hepatic metastases.**

False.

❏❏ **What is the typical clinical presentation of patients with benign lesions of the liver?**

They are most commonly discovered incidentally in the course of evaluation of unrelated symptoms.

❏❏ **What treatment options are available for patients with hepatic cysts?**

Observation, aspiration, sclerosis, various forms of internal drainage and resection.

❏❏ **What is the preferred treatment for patients with symptomatic adult polycystic liver disease?**

Resection combined with fenestration.

❏❏ **What organisms produce hydatid cysts of the liver?**

Echinococcus granulosus and Echinococcus multilocularis.

❏❏ **What factors are evaluated in Child's criteria for stratifying the severity of liver disease?**

Nutritional status, encephalopathy, ascites, serum bilirubin, serum albumin and prothrombin time.

❏❏ **What is the proper treatment for patients with bleeding gastric varices, without esophageal varices?**

Splenectomy.

❏❏ **What are the key issues in the management of patients with portal hypertension resulting from the Budd-Chiari syndrome?**

Patency of the IVC and the quality of liver function.

❏❏ **What is the composition of hepatic bile?**

Water and electrolytes (90%) and organic solutes (10%).

❏❏ **What are the diagnostic criteria for spontaneous bacterial peritonitis (SBP)?**

A history of cirrhosis (usually with ascites), abdominal pain, fever, increased WBC count and peritoneal fluid containing greater than 250 PMNs/mm3.

❏❏ **What is the appropriate treatment for patients with SBP?**

A third generation cephalosporin.

❐❐ What is the most important consideration in repair of hernias in patients with liver disease?

Presence of ascites.

❐❐ What is the advantage of a selective shunt over a nonselective shunt?

A selective shunt will preserve hepatic blood flow and reduce the risk of portosystemic encephalopathy.

❐❐ What is the first line of therapy for patients with bleeding esophageal varices?

Endoscopic banding or sclerotherapy.

❐❐ What is the risk of death from bleeding esophageal varices?

20 to 50%.

❐❐ What is the role of propranolol in the management of patients with bleeding esophageal varices?

It reduces the risk of rebleeding after a first bleed by decreasing the portal pressure.

❐❐ What pressure defines portal hypertension and why?

12 mm Hg is generally accepted as portal hypertension. Below this level, bleeding from varices is rarely seen.

❐❐ What substances are thought to be responsible for the hyperdynamic circulation seen in patients with cirrhosis and portal hypertension?

Prostaglandins, glucagon, nitric oxide and TNF.

❐❐ What arterial supply is shared by the head of the pancreas and the second and third portions of the duodenum, necessitating en bloc resection of the duodenum with lesions of the pancreatic head?

The inferior pancreaticoduodenal artery, from the superior mesenteric artery, collateralizes with the superior pancreaticoduodenal artery, arising from the gastroduodenal artery.

❐❐ What is the only pancreatic enzyme secreted in active form?

Amylase.

❐❐ Where is enterokinase located?

In the brush border of intestinal epithelial cells.

❐❐ What are the most frequent complications following major hepatic resection?

Hemorrhage and bile leak.

❐❐ What is the role of transjugular intrahepatic portosystemic shunting (TIPS) in the management of patients with variceal hemorrhage?

TIPS is a temporary shunt. It is most suited to the management of variceal hemorrhage in patients not responding to banding or sclerotherapy and those with gastric varices. It is an excellent bridge to transplantation for patients who might not tolerate a surgical shunt and who are candidates for liver transplantation.

❏❏ **What is Stage I Hodgkin's disease?**

One area, or two contiguous areas, of lymph node involvement on the same side of the diaphragm.

❏❏ **Which hemorrhagic disorder is characterized by destruction of platelets by circulating IgG antiplatelet antibodies?**

Idiopathic thrombocytopenia purpura (ITP).

❏❏ **What is the role of active and passive immunization for viral hepatitis?**

Vaccines are available for hepatitis A and B and are very effective. There is no vaccine for hepatitis C. Immunoglobulin (Ig) therapy is indicated for exposure to any form of hepatitis. Specific, effective Ig is available for hepatitis B. Passive immunization is recommended for accidental needle stick exposure for hepatitis B and C. Knowledge of the serologic status of the source is critical in guiding therapy.

❏❏ **What vessels are contained within the gastrosplenic ligament?**

The short gastrics.

❏❏ **What is the 5-year survival rate following pancreaticoduodenectomy for distal adenocarcinoma of the bile ducts?**

30%.

❏❏ **What is the most common location for an accessory spleen?**

At the hilus of the spleen.

❏❏ **What is the primary pathophysiology in acalculous cholecystitis?**

Gallbladder stasis.

❏❏ **What are the clinical features of hereditary spherocytosis?**

Anemia, reticulocytosis, jaundice and splenomegaly.

❏❏ **What is the most common type of thalassemia in the United States?**

Beta-thalassemia.

❏❏ **What type of anemia is associated with thalassemia major?**

A hypochromic, microcytic anemia.

❏❏ **What are the indications for surgical staging of Hodgkin's disease?**

Patients with clinical stage I and II disease and asymptomatic patients with the nodular sclerosing type.

❏❏ **What is Felty's syndrome?**

The triad of rheumatoid arthritis, splenomegaly and neutropenia.

❏❏ **What are the indications for splenectomy in a patient with Felty's syndrome?**

Recurrent infections with neutropenia, patients requiring transfusion for anemia, profound thrombocytopenia and intractable leg ulcers.

❑❑ **What is the embryologic origin of the spleen?**

Mesenchymal differentiation in the dorsal mesogastrum.

❑❑ **What is the most appropriate initial diagnostic test for a patient with obstructive jaundice?**

Ultrasonography.

❑❑ **What is the composition of the white pulp of the spleen?**

Lymphatic follicles and periarteriolar lymphatic sheets.

❑❑ **What is the primary function of the red pulp?**

Phagocytosis.

❑❑ **What is the primary function of the white pulp?**

Immunologic.

❑❑ **What are the normal splenic functions?**

It serves as a reservoir for circulating platelets, a blood filter for old/damaged RBCs, bacteria and particulate antigens, phagocytosis and production of tuftsin, antibodies (especially IgM), opsonins and properdin.

❑❑ **What familial disorder is characterized by abnormal storage of glycolipid cerebrosides in reticuloendothelial cells?**

Gaucher's disease.

❑❑ **What is the main chemical component of pigment gallstones?**

Calcium bilirubinate.

❑❑ **What are the common signs of pancreatitis?**

Fever, tachycardia, hypotension, a distended abdomen, guarding and diminished or absent bowel sounds. Rarely seen signs include tender subcutaneous nodules from fat necrosis and hypocalcemic tetany.

❑❑ **What is the most common parasitic cyst of the spleen?**

Echinoccus.

❑❑ **What is the most common tumor of the spleen?**

Sarcoma.

❑❑ **A 23 year old IV drug abuser presents to the emergency room with fever, chills, splenomegaly and left upper quadrant abdominal tenderness. What is the most likely diagnosis?**

A splenic abscess.

❑❑ **What is Kehr's sign?**

Pain at the tip of the shoulder, which is evidence of diaphragmatic irritation.

❑❑ **How often is Kehr's sign present in patients with a splenic injury?**

Less than 50% of the time.

❏❏ **What is the stimulus for release of pancreatic enzymes?**

Cholecystokinin and vagal cholinergics.

❏❏ **What is the gastric phase of pancreatic secretion?**

When food enters the stomach.

❏❏ **What are the indications for operation in patients with a splenic injury?**

Injuries to other intraabdominal organs, increasing peritoneal signs and evidence of continued bleeding.

❏❏ **Following splenectomy for trauma, what is the risk of overwhelming postsplenectomy sepsis in children? In adults?**

0.6% in children and 0.3% in adults.

❏❏ **What is the most common familial hemolytic anemia?**

Hereditary spherocytosis.

❏❏ **In 10% of normal people the embryologic dorsal and ventral pancreatic ducts do not fuse. What is this known as?**

Pancreas divisum.

❏❏ **What is the blood supply to the head of the pancreas?**

The superior pancreaticoduodenal artery.

❏❏ **How much fluid is secreted by the exocrine pancreas per day?**

1 to 2 liters.

❏❏ **What are the principle cations in pancreatic juice?**

Sodium and potassium.

❏❏ **What are the principle anions in pancreatic juice?**

Bicarbonate and chloride.

❏❏ **At what vertebral level will you find the head of the pancreas? The body? The tail?**

L2, L1 and T12, respectively.

❏❏ **What is the anatomic relationship of the uncinate process of the pancreas to the portal vein and superior mesenteric vessels?**

The uncinate process is posterior to the vessels.

❏❏ **What cells synthesize somatostatin?**

Delta cells.

❏❏ **What is the embryologic etiology of an annular pancreas?**

Abnormal rotation and fusion of the ventral pancreatic primordium.

❑❑ **What is the colon cut-off sign?**

A gas-filled ascending and right transverse colon that stops abruptly in the mid- or left transverse colon.

❑❑ **What is the significance of the colon cut-off sign?**

It is caused by inflammation of the pancreas, which induces spasm in the adjacent colon.

❑❑ **What is the most common cause of chronic pancreatitis in the United States?**

Alcoholism.

❑❑ **What is the most common location for an ectopic pancreas?**

In the stomach or duodenum.

❑❑ **What is the typical presentation of patients with acute pancreatitis?**

Severe and persistent epigastric or upper abdominal pain that often radiates to the back.

❑❑ **What is Cullen's sign?**

A bluish color around the umbilicus.

❑❑ **What is the most common cause of acute pancreatitis in the United States?**

Cholelithiasis.

❑❑ **What are the morphologic characteristics of the pancreas in patients with mild acute pancreatitis?**

Pancreatic and peripancreatic edema and fat necrosis.

❑❑ **What are the two most common causes of pancreatic pseudocysts?**

Alcohol abuse and biliary tract disease.

❑❑ **In what region of the pancreas do most pseudocysts occur?**

In the body.

❑❑ **What is the most sensitive and specific diagnostic test for pseudocysts?**

CT scan.

❑❑ **How long does it take for a pseudocyst to mature sufficiently enough for surgical resection?**

4 to 6 weeks (unless the cyst arises during acute pancreatitis, in which case no waiting is necessary).

❑❑ **What is the most common islet cell neoplasm?**

An insulinoma.

❑❑ **What is the classic diagnostic (Whipple's) triad for insulinomas?**

Hypoglycemic symptoms produced by fasting, blood glucose less than 50 mg/dl during symptomatic episodes and relief of symptoms with intravenous administration of glucose.

❏❏ **What percentage of patients who undergo external drainage of a pancreatic pseudocyst will develop a pancreatic fistula?**

20%.

❏❏ **What is Courvoisier's sign and what does its presence suggest?**

It is a distended and palpable gallbladder in a jaundiced patient. It suggests malignant obstruction.

❏❏ **What characteristic finding on ERCP suggests pancreatic cancer?**

Constriction of the pancreatic and bile ducts in the head of the gland (the double duct sign).

❏❏ **What organs are resected in the Whipple procedure?**

The distal stomach, gallbladder, common bile duct, head of the pancreas, duodenum, proximal jejunum and regional lymphatics.

❏❏ **What is the etiology of Zollinger-Ellison syndrome?**

Gastric acid hypersecretion caused by excessive gastrin production.

❏❏ **What areas of the pancreas are usually drained by the duct of Santorini?**

The anterior and posterior portions of the head.

❏❏ **What is the stimulus for secretion of pancreatic juice?**

Secretin (released from the duodenum and proximal small bowel in response to acid).

❏❏ **What is the effect of somatostatin on pancreatic secretion?**

It is inhibitory.

❏❏ **T/F: Lithocholic acid is a primary bile salt.**

False.

❏❏ **Where do most gastrinomas occur?**

In the pancreas.

❏❏ **What percentage of gastrinomas are non-beta islet cell carcinomas?**

60%.

❏❏ **What percentage of gastrinomas are associated with the MEN-1 syndrome?**

25%.

❏❏ **What are the most common symptoms of gastrinoma?**

Severe, refractory peptic ulcer disease and diarrhea.

❏❏ **What are the typical manifestations of WDHA?**

Profuse watery diarrhea with loss of large amounts of potassium; hypokalemia, profound weakness, severe metabolic acidosis and hypercalcemia.

❒❒ **What is the typical constellation of symptoms seen in patients with glucagonomas?**

Migratory necrolytic dermatitis, weight loss, stomatitis, hypoaminoacidemia and mild diabetes.

❒❒ **What are the functions of the acinar cells of the pancreas?**

They produce and secrete digestive enzymes.

❒❒ **What do the ductal cells of the pancreas produce?**

Bicarbonate.

❒❒ **What is the second most common cause of chronic pancreatitis?**

Idiopathic.

❒❒ **What are the characteristic histologic findings of chronic pancreatitis?**

Loss of exocrine acinar cells, a marked increase in interstitial connective tissue, hyperplasia of the islet cells and perineural sheath damage.

❒❒ **What is the most common complication of acute pancreatitis?**

Pseudocyst formation.

❒❒ **What is the primary indication for hepatic resection in cirrhotic patients?**

Hepatocellular carcinoma.

❒❒ **What are the indications for surgical drainage of a pancreatic pseudocyst?**

A persistently symptomatic (i.e., pain, anorexia and biliary or gastrointestinal obstruction), an enlarging pseudocyst and onset of a pseudocyst complication.

❒❒ **T/F: Cigarette smoking is the most strongly associated risk factor for adenocarcinoma of the pancreas.**

True.

❒❒ **Glycolysis generates how many molecules of ATP for each molecule of glucose?**

37; with 1 molecule reserved for storage.

❒❒ **T/F: The falciform ligament demarcates the right hepatic lobe from the left hepatic lobe.**

False.

❒❒ **When performing complex biliary procedures, where in the hepatoduodenal ligament would you expect to find the common bile duct?**

The duct is most lateral with the hepatic artery medial and the portal vein most posterior.

❒❒ **A 36 year old otherwise healthy female undergoes a left hepatic lobectomy for a large adenoma. A cholecystectomy is performed concurrently, despite a negative history of cholelithiasis** or any intraoperative indications of cholecystitis. What is the rationale for including a cholecystectomy with this resection?

Anatomically, the left lobe of the live extends to the gallbladder fossa. Upon resection of the left lobe, the line of devascularization demarcates in this area, necessitating a cholecystectomy.

❏❏ **What are the most common causative organisms for a pyogenic hepatic abscess?**

Enteric bacteria (gram negative facultative aerobic rods, streptococci and Bacteroides fragilis).

❏❏ **What is the most common cause of portal hypertension in the US?**

Cirrhosis, most frequently due to alcoholism.

❏❏ **What is the most common cause of portal hypertension world-wide?**

Schistosomiasis.

❏❏ **What is the pathophysiology leading to portal hypertension in patients with cirrhosis?**

Postsinusoidal fibrosis in the Space of Disse and hepatic venous distortion due to nodular formation.

❏❏ **A 65 year old chronic alcoholic with a known history of cirrhosis presents with a slight increase in abdominal girth and mental status changes consistent with grade II encephalopathy. Laboratory evaluation reveals a serum albumin of 3.0 gm/dl, a total bilirubin of 3.1 mg/dl and a PT of 4.0 sec. What is his Child-Pugh classification?**

Child's B.

❏❏ **T/F: Hepatorenal syndrome is characterized by decreased urine sodium.**

True.

❏❏ **What is the frequency of SBP in cirrhotic patients with ascites?**

10%.

❏❏ **What is the drug of choice for patients with hepatic encephalopathy?**

Neomycin. Lactulose is also used, as it acidifies the colonic lumen and maintains ammonia in the ionized state.

❏❏ **In evaluating ascitic fluid obtained from a patient presumed to have SBP, what laboratory findings are expected?**

A WBC count greater than 500/μl with greater than 25% PMNs, a serum albumin:ascitic fluid albumin gradient greater than 1.1 gm/dl, a serum lactic acid level greater than 33 mg/dl and an ascitic fluid pH of less than 7.31.

❏❏ **What is the natural history of SBP given appropriate medical therapy?**

50% resolve (but 50% of these recur).

❏❏ **What is the treatment of choice for patients with hepatocellular adenomas?**

Surgical excision (usually lobectomy).

❏❏ **What is the approximate length of the common bile duct?**

7 to 9 cms.

❑❑ **What is the most common origin of the cystic artery?**

The right hepatic artery.

❑❑ **T/F: Muscularis mucosal and submucosal layers exist in the wall of the gallbladder.**

False.

❑❑ **What volume of bile is generated daily?**

About 1 liter.

❑❑ **What factors are responsible for the regulation of bile flow?**

The rate of hepatic secretion of bile, gallbladder contraction and sphincteric resistance at the ampulla.

❑❑ **Which gastrointestinal hormone is the major stimulus of gallbladder contraction and sphincter relaxation?**

Cholecystokinin.

❑❑ **How efficient is enterohepatic recirculation in maintaining the bile salt pool?**

95%.

❑❑ **A patient's main presenting complaint is diarrhea. Which neuroendocrine tumors of the pancreas are commonly associated with this symptom?**

Gastrinoma, VIPoma and somatostatinoma.

❑❑ **If a patient is referred to you for possible insulinoma and the insulin levels are normal or elevated, how can factitious hypoglycemia be ruled out?**

C-peptide level determination.

❑❑ **Why is preoperative localization of an insulinoma important?**

Most of these tumors are small and there is uniform distribution throughout the gland.

❑❑ **What laboratory value is helpful in distinguishing an elevated level of alkaline phosphatase due to bone disease and that due to hepatobiliary pathology?**

5'-nucleotidase.

❑❑ **T/F: The majority of gallstones in the United States are cholesterol stones.**

True.

❑❑ **What is the efficacy of ultrasound in positively identifying gallstones?**

About 95%.

SMALL INTESTINE, COLON, RECTUM AND ANUS PEARLS

Hypochondria is the only disease I haven't got.
Anonymous

❑❑ **What is Denonvillier's fascia?**

The rectovesical septum in men and the rectovaginal septum in women.

❑❑ **What are the contents of the ischiorectal fossa?**

The inferior rectal vessels and lymphatics.

❑❑ **What is the treatment of choice for a patient with a perirectal abscess?**

Surgical drainage.

❑❑ **What is the etiology of rectoceles in women?**

Weakened muscle and soft tissue between the rectum and vagina after years of straining to defecate.

❑❑ **In which region of the colon does volvulus most frequently occur?**

The sigmoid colon.

❑❑ **What is the etiology of a cecal volvulus?**

Anomalous fixation of the right colon to the retroperitoneum.

❑❑ **What is the most common form of gastrointestinal ischemia?**

Ischemic colitis.

❑❑ **What are the characteristic symptoms of anal fissures?**

Tearing pain on defecation, blood on the toilet paper or stool and, rarely, blood in the toilet bowl.

❑❑ **A 41 year old female presents with a history of a chronic anal lesion unresponsive to conservative management. Physical examination reveals an anal fissure in the posterior midline, a sentinel skin tag and hypertrophied anal papilla. What is the treatment of choice?**

A lateral internal sphincterotomy.

❑❑ **A 38 year old male presents with a history of painless, bright red rectal bleeding associated with bowel movements. What is the most likely diagnosis?**

Internal hemorrhoids.

❑❑ **What is the most appropriate treatment for first and second degree hemorrhoids?**

Increase dietary fiber, stool softeners and avoidance of straining at stool.

❏❏ **What is the anatomic distinction between internal and external hemorrhoids?**

Internal hemorrhoids occur above the dentate line, external hemorrhoids occur below it.

❏❏ **Where is a low rectovaginal fistula located?**

Close to the dentate line, with the vaginal opening just inside the fourchette.

❏❏ **What is the relationship of pilonidal cysts to the postsacral fascia?**

Pilonidal cysts are superficial to the postsacral fascia.

❏❏ **What is the usual location of a pilonidal cyst if the external orifice is visible?**

In the midline, approximately 5 cm from the anus.

❏❏ **What is hidradenitis suppurativa?**

An infection of the cutaneous apocrine sweat glands.

❏❏ **What organism causes chancroid?**

Haemophilus ducreyi.

❏❏ **What is the treatment of choice for chancroid?**

Sulfonamides.

❏❏ **What are the secondary lesions of syphilis?**

Condyloma lata.

❏❏ **What is the most common means of transmission of Condylomata acuminata?**

Anal intercourse.

❏❏ **What is the appropriate treatment for patients with small condyloma warts?**

Bichloracetic acid and 25% podophyllin.

❏❏ **Which of the human papilloma viruses (HPV) are associated with carcinoma of the anal and genital tracts?**

HPV 16 and 18.

❏❏ **What is the most common cause of mesenteric ischemia?**

Superior mesenteric artery (SMA) embolism.

❏❏ **What is primary mesenteric venous thrombosis?**

Spontaneous occlusion of the mesenteric veins, without trauma or co-existing hematologic, liver or cardiac disease.

❏❏ **What is the arterial blood supply to the colon and rectum?**

The superior mesenteric, inferior mesenteric and hypogastric arteries.

❑❑ **What is the most common presentation of intestinal ischemia?**

Abdominal pain out of proportion to physical findings.

❑❑ **What are the angiographic criteria for non-occlusive mesenteric ischemia?**

Narrowing at the origins of major SMA branches, irregularities of distal branches, with alternating dilatation and constriction, spasm of peripheral arcades and impaired filling of intramural vessels.

❑❑ **What is the treatment of choice for a patient with non-occlusive mesenteric ischemia without peritonitis?**

Intraarterial infusion of papaverine.

❑❑ **What is the usual cause of pseudomembranous colitis?**

Antibiotic therapy.

❑❑ **What is the most common protozoon that infects the colon?**

E. histolytica.

❑❑ **Which recreational drug has been associated with ischemic colitis?**

Cocaine.

❑❑ **What percentage of patients with AIDS develop cytomegalovirus (CMV) colitis?**

90%.

❑❑ **What is the etiology of Chaga's disease?**

Trypanosoma cruzi.

❑❑ **What diagnostic tests are most sensitive for mesenteric venous thrombosis?**

CT scan and MRI.

❑❑ **Which blood vessel is the most important collateral to the left colon?**

The marginal artery of Drummond.

❑❑ **What is the most common source of arterial emboli to the SMA?**

The left atrium.

❑❑ **The celiac trunk courses anteriorly for a short distance inferior to which structure?**

The arcuate ligament of the diaphragm.

❑❑ **What is the success rate of percutaneous transluminal angioplasty (PTA) for chronic mesenteric ischemia?**

80 to 90%.

❑❑ **Reperfusion injury is due at least in part to the cytotoxic effect of which class of compounds?**

Reactive oxygen species (ROS).

❑❑ **Non-occlusive mesenteric ischemia accounts for approximately what percentage of all cases of mesenteric ischemia?**

20%.

❑❑ **If isolated right colon ischemia is found, what should be the next diagnostic test?**

Mesenteric arteriography.

❑❑ **What is the venous drainage of the distal rectum?**

The inferior hemorrhoidal vein, which drains into the iliac vein.

❑❑ **What is the most common splanchnic artery aneurysm?**

Splenic artery aneurysm.

❑❑ **What classifications of drugs are often associated with non-occlusive mesenteric ischemia?**

Vasopressors and alpha-adrenergic agonists.

❑❑ **What is the most reliable way to make the diagnosis of colonic ischemia?**

Flexible sigmoidoscopy or colonoscopy.

❑❑ **Under resting states, which layer of the bowel receives the majority of total intestinal blood flow?**

The mucosa receives between 50 to 65% of intestinal blood flow at rest.

❑❑ **What is the sine qua non of intestinal ischemia?**

Tissue hypoxia.

❑❑ **What is the most common vascular malformation of the gastrointestinal tract?**

Angiodysplasia.

❑❑ **What is the name of the small bowel mucosa characterized by transverse folds?**

The valves of Kerckring (valvulae circulares).

❑❑ **What is the strongest component of the small bowel wall?**

The submucosa.

❑❑ **What nerve plexus lies within the submucosa of the small intestine?**

Meissner's plexus.

❑❑ **Where are bile salts reabsorbed?**

In the ileum.

❑❑ **What is the optimal form for protein for absorption in the small intestine?**

Peptides, 2 to 6 amino acids long.

❑❑ **T/F: Glucose absorption in the small intestine occurs by facilitated diffusion.**

False.

❑❑ **What is the net amount of fluid, not reabsorbed in the small intestine, that passes into the colon?**

Approximately 0.5 l/day.

❑❑ **Which small intestinal hormone is released by acidification or bile contact in the duodenal mucosa and results in release of water and bicarbonate from pancreatic ductal cells?**

Secretin.

❑❑ **Which gut hormone is released from the small bowel mucosa after contact with tryptophan and/or fatty acids and results in secretion of enzymes by pancreatic acinar cells?**

Cholecystokinin.

❑❑ **Which gut hormone is capable of contraction of intestinal smooth muscle and plays a significant role in controlling the interdigestive pattern of gut motility?**

Motilin.

❑❑ **What is the major immunoglobulin secreted from cells in the lamina propria of the small intestine?**

IgA.

❑❑ **What is bacterial translocation?**

Passage of viable bacteria from the intact gastrointestinal tract lumen to mesenteric lymph nodes and, possibly, the liver. Small intestinal integrity is impaired as a result of a variety of systemic injuries.

❑❑ **How can bacterial translocation be decreased?**

By enteral feeding.

❑❑ **What are the two most important pathologic characteristics of Crohn's disease of the small intestine?**

Transmural inflammation and the presence of noncaseating granulomas with Langerhan's giant cells.

❑❑ **A 22 year old male with a suspected appendicitis is undergoing right lower quadrant exploration. The appendix is found to be normal and further exploration reveals obvious Crohn's disease of the terminal ileum. What is the treatment of choice?**

Appendectomy if the cecum is grossly clear of disease.

❑❑ **T/F: Enterocutaneous fistulas usually occur spontaneously in patients with Crohn's disease.**

False.

❑❑ **What is the most common primary small bowel malignancy?**

Adenocarcinoma.

❏❏ **Where are benign adenomas of the small intestine most commonly located?**

In the ileum.

❏❏ **The characteristic soap bubble appearance on contrast radiography, of a lesion in the duodenum, is consistent with what diagnosis?**

Villous adenoma of the duodenum.

❏❏ **What is Peutz-Jeghers syndrome?**

A Mendelian dominant, inherited syndrome consisting of mucocutaneous melanotic pigmentation and multiple gastrointestinal polyps.

❏❏ **T/F: The gastrointestinal polyps associated with Peutz-Jeghers syndrome are premalignant.**

False.

❏❏ **What are the most common complications of juvenile polyposis?**

Gastrointestinal bleeding and obstruction.

❏❏ **What are the histological characteristics of hyperplastic polyps?**

Epithelial dysmaturation and hyperplasia.

❏❏ **T/F: Polypectomy decreases the risk of colon carcinoma.**

True.

❏❏ **What is Cowden's syndrome?**

An autosomal dominant defect that includes hamartomas of all 3 embryonal cell layers.

❏❏ **Leiomyosarcomas of the small intestine metastasize most frequently by what mechanism?**

Hematogenous dissemination.

❏❏ **What is the Lynch syndrome?**

Inherited nonpolyposis colon cancer.

❏❏ **What is the most frequent site of intestinal carcinoid tumors?**

The appendix (46%, followed by ileum at 28%).

❏❏ **What percentage of ileal carcinoids are associated with metastatic disease?**

35%.

❏❏ **What is the most common small intestine location for diverticular formation?**

The duodenum.

❏❏ **What is the rule of two's for Meckel's diverticulum?**

Meckel's diverticulum occurs in 2% of the population, generally within 2 feet of the ileocecal valve, may contain 2 types of heterotopic tissue (gastric or pancreatic) and the incidence of symptomatic Meckel's diverticulum is 2%.

❏❏ **T/F: Incidental removal of an asymptomatic Meckel's diverticulum is associated with a decreased risk of developing complications.**

False.

❏❏ **T/F: Pneumatosis cystoides intestinalis is usually a primary pathologic process in the jejunum.**

False.

❏❏ **What vitamin deficiency occurs most frequently in patients with a significant blind loop syndrome?**

B12 deficiency, due to bacterial competition for the vitamin.

❏❏ **What diagnostic test is performed to confirm blind loop syndrome as the cause of B12 deficiency?**

A Schilling test, in which increased B12 absorption occurs after the administration of oral tetracycline for 3 to 5 days.

❏❏ **What is the predominant source of gaseous distention in cases of small bowel obstruction?**

Swallowed air.

❏❏ **What is the definition of strangulation obstruction?**

An obstructed segment of small intestine that has compromised tissue blood flow resulting in necrosis and gangrene.

❏❏ **What type of flora dominates the normal distal ileum?**

Anaerobic organisms.

❏❏ **What is the source of short-chain fatty acids that serve as an important energy supply for colonocytes?**

Metabolism of fecal sterols by intestinal bacteria.

❏❏ **What is the definition of cecal distention?**

A diameter greater than 10 cm.

❏❏ **What percentage of small bowel obstructions, secondary to operative adhesions, resolve nonoperatively?**

80%.

❏❏ **What is the treatment of choice for patients with gallstone ileus?**

Identification of the impacted gallstone in the small bowel followed by a proximal enterotomy with retrieval of the gallstone. Cholecystectomy should not be performed at the initial operation.

☐☐ **T/F: Small bowel obstruction in patients with a previous malignancy is related to operative adhesions in 50% of cases.**

True.

☐☐ **The highest incidence of Crohn's disease occurs in what population?**

Ashkenazi Jews born outside of Israel. Jewish people are afflicted 3 to 8 times more often than non-Jews. Ashkenazi Jews born outside of Israel have a 4-fold increase in the disease compared to Ashkenazi Jews born in Israel.

☐☐ **T/F: There is an increased incidence of Crohn's disease in first and second generation relatives of patients with Crohn's disease.**

True.

☐☐ **What is the most frequent site of gastrointestinal Crohn's disease?**

The ileocecal region, which accounts for approximately 50% of cases.

☐☐ **What percentage of patients with Crohn's disease demonstrate noncaseating granulomas?**

66%.

☐☐ **What is the mechanism for the increased incidence of oxalate stones in patients with extensive Crohn's disease of the terminal ileum?**

Increased intestinal water loss and a lack of unchelated intraluminal calcium secondary to fatty acid saponification, which enables free oxalate to reach the colon, where it is absorbed.

☐☐ **Crohn's disease in what area of the GI tract is most commonly associated with perianal disease?**

In the ileocolic region.

☐☐ **What is the most common type of intestinal fistula seen in patients with Crohn's disease?**

Enteroenteric.

☐☐ **T/F: TPN is superior to enteral diets in achieving remission of small intestinal Crohn's disease.**

False.

☐☐ **What is the active component of sulfasalazine in the management of Crohn's disease and ulcerative colitis?**

The 5-ASA moiety.

☐☐ **What are the three types of small intestinal adenomas?**

Tubular, villous and Brunner gland adenomas.

☐☐ **Which type of small intestine adenoma has the greatest malignant potential?**

Villous adenomas.

☐☐ **What disease is associated with multiple familial angiomatoses of the gastrointestinal tract?**

Osler-Weber-Rendu disease.

❑❑ **What is the most common location for villous adenomas of the small intestine?**

The duodenum.

❑❑ **What is the most common primary malignancy that spreads hematogenously to the small intestine?**

Malignant melanoma.

❑❑ **What are the most common etiologies of ileus?**

Postoperative, peritonitis and hypokalemia.

❑❑ **In what order do the stomach, small intestine and colon resume normal motility following intraabdominal procedures?**

The small intestine returns within 24 hours, the stomach in 24 to 48 hours and the colon in 40 to 48 hours.

❑❑ **T/F: Reglan stimulates colonic motility.**

False.

❑❑ **What organism is most frequently seen in bacterial overgrowth of the small bowel, in the presence of obstruction?**

Bacteroides.

❑❑ **What are the most common etiologies of intestinal obstruction in the United States?**

Adhesions, followed by hernias and neoplasms.

❑❑ **T/F: Barium enema is the treatment of choice for reduction of intussception in adults.**

False.

❑❑ **After 8 weeks in an external fixator for a complex pelvic fracture, the device is removed. The patient subsequently experiences severe abdominal pain upon lying supine. The pain is only relieved in the knee-to-chest position. What is the most likely diagnosis?**

SMA syndrome.

❑❑ **Why is there a decreased incidence of small intestinal carcinomas compared to other portions of the GI tract?**

The small bowel has a rapid transit time (1 to 2 hours), decreased exposure to potential carcinogens, an alkaline pH, decreased bacterial growth and elevated levels of benzopyrene hydroxylase, an enzyme that detoxifies possible carcinogens.

❑❑ **What extraintestinal manifestations are associated with familial adenomatous polyposis (FAP)?**

Epidermoid cysts, dermoid tumors of the abdomen, osteomas and brain tumors (usually gliomas and medulloblastomas).

❑❑ **What is the inheritance pattern of FAP?**

Autosomal dominant.

❑❑ **What percentage of patients with untreated FAP develop colon cancer?**

100%.

❑❑ **What is Turcot's syndrome?**

Colonic polyps and glioma or medulloblastoma.

❑❑ **What are the dietary recommendations by the National Resource Council to decrease the risk of developing colorectal carcinoma?**

1. Dietary fat should not exceed 30% of total calories.
2. Increase consumption of fiber-containing foods.
3. Limit salt-cured, pickled and smoked foods.
4. Limit food additives shown to be carcinogenic.
5. Limit alcohol consumption.

❑❑ **What is the procedure of choice for a patient with carcinoma in the right colon?**

A right hemicolectomy, including 10 cm of terminal ileum, with ligation of the ileocolic artery, right colic artery and the right branch of the middle colic artery.

❑❑ **What margins of resection are required for colon carcinoma?**

5 cm is ideal, however, 2 cm may be adequate.

❑❑ **What is the 5-year survival rate for patients with Stage II colon carcinoma?**

60 to 80%.

❑❑ **What is the procedure of choice for patients with rectal carcinoma, in whom the sphincter mechanism cannot be preserved?**

Abdominal perineal resection (APR).

❑❑ **What is the incidence of malignancy in patients with large villous polyps?**

30%.

❑❑ **What is the most common benign tumor of the small intestine?**

Leiomyoma.

❑❑ **Where do the majority of duodenal malignancies occur?**

In the periampullary region.

❑❑ **What is the role of surgery in intestinal lymphoma?**

For staging (liver biopsies and paraaortic and mesenteric lymph node sampling).

❑❑ **What age group is most often affected with Crohn's disease?**

There are 2 peaks, 15 to 30 years old and 50 to 60 years old.

❑❑ **What clinical triad is characteristic of Crohn's disease?**

Abdominal pain, diarrhea and weight loss.

❏❏ **How does a truncal vagotomy affect gastric emptying?**

Since the proximal and distal stomach is denervated, there is an increased rate of gastric emptying of liquids and solids.

❏❏ **A 21 year old female presents with chronic right lower quadrant pain and diarrhea. Her history is significant for Crohn's disease. What is the most likely diagnosis?**

Small bowel obstruction.

❏❏ **What percentage of patients with Crohn's disease proceed to toxic megacolon?**

6%.

❏❏ **What are the characteristics of toxic megacolon?**

Submucosal inflammation, destruction of the muscularis propria and myenteric plexus, atony and distention. It may be precipitated by analgesics, antidiarrheals and anticholinergics, all routine therapies for patients with this disease.

❏❏ **What features of Crohn's disease are seen on colonoscopy?**

Linear ulcerations, cobble-stoning, asymmetric involvement, skip lesions and apthous ulcers.

❏❏ **What surgical principles apply to intervention for complications of Crohn's disease?**

Thorough exploration for skip lesions, conservative resection, margins need not be microscopically negative and frozen sections are not necessary. If tissues appear grossly normal, anastomosis is appropriate and safe.

❏❏ **What are the two types of neural plexusus found in the colon?**

The submucosal (Meissner's) and the myenteric (Auerbach's) plexuses.

❏❏ **What percentage of patients with diverticulitis have a tender abdominal mass?**

20% (it portends a poorer prognosis).

❏❏ **What is the etiology of diverticula?**

Diverticula form at weak points, consisting of sites at which the vasa recta penetrate the circular muscle layer en route to the mucosa.

❏❏ **An 82 year old nursing home patient with Alzheimer's disease presents with a 24-hour history of severe abdominal distention, without significant pain or tenderness. Abdominal x-rays reveal a large, air-filled right colon. What is the most likely diagnosis?**

Ogilvie's syndrome.

❏❏ **What are the most common causes of massive colonic bleeding?**

Diverticulosis and angiodysplasia.

❏❏ **Which part of the colon is most likely to be involved in hemorrhage from diverticulosis?**

The right colon (70 to 90%).

❏❏ In patients who present with confirmed diverticular bleeding, what percentage cease bleeding spontaneously?

70%.

❏❏ What is the differential diagnosis in a 75 year old male with mild to moderate, intermittent lower abdominal pain?

Chronic constipation, diverticulosis, diverticulitis, ischemic colitis, irritable bowel syndrome and adenocarcinoma of the colon.

❏❏ A 50 year old male presents with melena. What rate of hemorrhage is required to detect the source of bleeding by selective angiography?

0.5 to 1 ml/min.

❏❏ A 50 year old patient presents with his second episode of lower GI bleeding from diverticulosis, localized by colonoscopy to the sigmoid. What is the treatment of choice?

After controlling the hemorrhage, a sigmoid colectomy should be performed. 25% of patients with initial diverticular bleeding have a recurrence and most patients continue to have recurrences without surgical intervention.

❏❏ What is backwash ileitis?

Mild inflammation and dilatation of the terminal ileum in patients with ulcerative colitis.

❏❏ What is the typical presentation of a patient with ulcerative colitis?

Bloody diarrhea, fever and abdominal pain.

❏❏ What percentage of patients with ulcerative colitis present total colonic involvement (pancolitis)?

10%.

❏❏ What characteristics of colonic polyps increase the malignant potential?

Size greater than 1 cm, villous-type adenoma, dysplasia and ulceration.

❏❏ What are the extraintestinal manifestations of ulcerative colitis?

Uveitis, iritis, episcleritis, keratitis, conjunctivitis, peripheral joint disease, arthralgias with progressive edema and erythema, ankylosing spondylitis, sacroiliitis, apthous stomatitis, gingivitis, pyoderma gangrenosum and sclerosing cholangitis.

❏❏ What is the Hartmann procedure?

Resection of the left and/or sigmoid colon with the creation of an end colostomy and closure of the distal defractionalized portion of the colon or rectum.

❏❏ What are the most common postoperative complaints following total proctocolectomy and ileoanal anastomosis?

Poor stool consistency, increased stool frequency and nocturnal stool leakage.

❏❏ **T/F: Preoperative counseling for patients undergoing a total proctocolectomy, with ileoanal anastomosis, should include advising the patient of the 10 to 25% incidence of small bowel obstruction.**

True.

❏❏ **On routine screening colonoscopy, a 68 year old female is found to have a 1 cm polyp at the splenic flexure. What is the most likely diagnosis?**

A tubular adenoma (77% of colorectal polyps 1 cm or less).

INTRAABDOMINAL INFECTIONS AND SURGICAL COMPLICATIONS PEARLS

The abdomen is the reason why man does not easily take himself for a god.
Freidrich Nietzsche

❏❏ **What is the most common source of bacteria in postoperative surgical infections?**

The patient.

❏❏ **What is the most common cause of intraabdominal compartment syndrome?**

Coagulopathy with postoperative intraabdominal hemorrhage.

❏❏ **What constitutes adequate tetanus immunization in an adult patient?**

3 injections of toxoid followed by a routine booster of adsorbed toxoid every 10 years.

❏❏ **What is the most common cause of fascial dehiscence?**

Intraabdominal sepsis.

❏❏ **What is the relationship between hepatitis B and D?**

Hepatitis D is an RNA virus coated with HBsAg as the surface protein. Infection with Hepatitis D can only occur as a co-infection with hepatitis B or as a superinfection in a hepatitis B carrier.

❏❏ **What is the most common viral pathogen complicating organ transplantation?**

Cytomegalovirus virus (CMV).

❏❏ **When is tetanus immune globulin (TIG) indicated?**

For patients with dirty wounds and for those who have not been previously vaccinated.

❏❏ **T/F: Pneumocystis carinii pneumonia (PCP) occurs only in HIV infected patients.**

False. There is a risk of PCP in any immunocompromised patient.

❏❏ **What is the latency period for seroconversion following exposure to the HIV virus?**

6 to 12 months.

❏❏ **Transmission of HIV infection in the workplace involves which body fluids?**

Saliva, stool, nasal secretions, sputum, tears, urine, sweat and vomitus.

❏❏ What are the common radiographic signs suggestive of esophageal perforation?

Mediastinal air, pneumothorax, pleural effusion, infiltrates and subcutaneous emphysema.

❏❏ T/F: Preoperative prophylactic antibiotics are indicated for patients undergoing an operation for gastric outlet obstruction.

True.

❏❏ A 31 year old multiple trauma patient develops bright red upper gastrointestinal bleeding on SICU day 6. What is the next step in management?

Upper endoscopy to identify the source of bleeding.

❏❏ What is the treatment of choice for patients with clostridium difficile colitis?

Oral metronidazole or vancomycin. For patients with severe ileus, intravenous metronidazole and vancomycin enemas may have some merit.

❏❏ When should prophylactic antibiotics be discontinued?

Within 12 hours after the operation. In many instances they may be discontinued at the end of the procedure.

❏❏ Why are iodine solutions superior to chlorhexidine as a surgical antiseptic?

Chlorhexidine is not effective against viruses and fungi.

❏❏ What systemic factors predispose a patient to wound infection?

Chronic granulomatous disease, renal failure, diabetes mellitus, malnutrition and immunosuppression.

❏❏ What is the best time to begin prophylactic antibiotic therapy for elective surgery?

1-2 hours prior to the operation.

❏❏ What is the best technique for removal of hair from the operative site?

Hair clipping.

❏❏ Excessive production and release of cytokines in the systemic inflammatory response initiates a cascade of events leading to organ failure. What are the triggering cells for this response?

Tissue macrophages.

❏❏ How long should antibiotics be continued for patients with an intraabdominal infection?

10 days.

❏❏ T/F: The etiology of the systemic inflammatory response is always infectious in origin.

False. Noninfectious causes of this syndrome include pancreatitis, ischemia, trauma, tissue injury, hemorrhagic shock and immune-mediated organ injury.

❏❏ What is the toxic portion of the endotoxin lipopolysaccharide protein complex?

Lipid A.

❏❏ **What factors can impair phagocytosis of bacteria?**

Bacterial encapsulation, uremia, prematurity, leukemia and hyperglycemia.

❏❏ **What pyrogen is responsible for raising the body temperature in response to infection?**

Interleukin-1.

❏❏ **What is the initial response to peritonitis?**

Vascular dilatation and fluid transudation.

❏❏ **What are the criteria for diagnosis of spontaneous bacterial peritonitis?**

An ascitic fluid neutrophil count of 250 cells/mm3, a positive ascitic fluid culture and the lack of an obvious intraabdominal source of infection.

❏❏ **What is the most common cause of pyuria associated with gross hematuria but without bacteriuria?**

Tuberculosis of the kidney.

❏❏ **In patients with postoperative pneumonia, empiric monotherapy should cover which organisms?**

Gram negative organisms.

❏❏ **T/F: Closed suction drainage decreases the incidence of wound infection in clean cases.**

False.

❏❏ **What are the most common organisms found in diabetic foot infections?**

Anaerobes.

❏❏ **Which antibiotics inhibit bacterial protein synthesis by binding reversibly to the 50S ribosomal subunit?**

Chloramphenicol, clindamycin and erythromycin.

❏❏ **T/F: Acute suppurative peritonitis is most commonly caused by a polymicrobial infection.**

True.

❏❏ **What local wound factors predispose patients to wound infections?**

Necrotic tissue, poor oxygenation, retained foreign body and undrained hematoma or seroma.

❏❏ **What is the most important factor in prevention of infection in diabetic patients?**

Control of diabetes.

❏❏ **What are the most common organisms cultured from pancreatic abscesses?**

Enteric organisms.

❏❏ **What are the most common causes of pelvic abscesses?**

A ruptured colonic diverticulum, pelvic inflammatory disease, a ruptured appendix or following resolution of a generalized peritonitis with pelvic drainage.

❏❏ **What are some of the considerations in choosing an antibiotic?**

Source and severity of the infection, patient age, renal impairment and local formulary considerations.

❏❏ **What type of peritonitis is caused by reactivation of a latent peritoneal tuberculous infection?**

Granulomatous peritonitis.

❏❏ **Penicillin is not active against which important anaerobic bacteria?**

Bacteroides fragilis.

❏❏ **What is the best test for localizing an intraabdominal abscess?**

CT scan.

❏❏ **What is the most common organism cultured from patients with the post-splenectomy sepsis syndrome?**

Streptococcus pneumonia.

❏❏ **Which antibiotic agents are bactericidal?**

Aminoglycosides, aztreonam, bacitracin, cephalosporins, imipenem, penicillins, polymyxins, quinolones and vancomycin.

❏❏ **What patient factors are associated with an increased risk of postoperative wound infection?**

Extremes of age, malnutrition, obesity, diabetes mellitus, hypoxemia, remote infection, corticosteroid therapy, recent operation, chronic inflammation and prior site irradiation.

❏❏ **T/F: Resistant organisms emerging in a patient during treatment with prophylactic antibiotics are associated with an increased risk of infection.**

True.

❏❏ **What is the incidence of wound infection in clean, clean-contaminated, contaminated and dirty cases?**

Less than 2, 10, 20 and 40%, respectively.

❏❏ **What classes of antibiotics inhibit bacterial protein synthesis by irreversibly binding to the 30S ribosomal subunit?**

Aminogycosides and tetracyclines.

❏❏ **Aztreonam belong to which class of antibiotics?**

The monobactams (monocyclic beta-lactam antibiotics).

❏❏ **What is the mechanism of acquiring Clostridium difficile colitis within the hospital?**

Person to person spread through a variety of routes, including direct patient-to-patient contact, transmission between patients from the hands of hospital personnel and contamination of medical instruments by an infected patient.

❏❏ **What are the important perioperative factors related to an increased risk of postoperative wound infection?**

Long preoperative hospitalization, no preoperative shower, early shaving of site, hair removal and prior antibiotic therapy.

❏❏ **What is the treatment of choice for a patient with tetanus?**

Excision and debridement of the wound, control of convulsions, antibiotics and 3000 to 6000 units of human tetanus immune globulin.

ABDOMINAL WALL, OMENTUM, MESENTARY AND RETROPERITONEUM PEARLS

The young physician starts life with twenty drugs for each disease.
The old physician ends life with one drug for twenty diseases.
William Osler

❏❏ **What is the blood supply to the anterior abdominal wall?**

The superior and inferior epigastric arteries, the lower intercostal arteries and the lumbar and circumflex iliac arteries.

❏❏ **Where do the lymphatics of the upper half of the abdominal wall drain?**

To the axillary nodes.

❏❏ **What are the components of the anterior rectus sheath?**

The external and internal oblique fascia.

❏❏ **What is the composition of the posterior rectus sheath above the linea semicircularis?**

A leaf of internal oblique fascia and transversalis fascia.

❏❏ **What is the most common location for malignant mesenteric tumors?**

At the root of the mesentery.

❏❏ **What is the most common solid omental tumor?**

Metastatic carcinoma.

❏❏ **What are the clinical characteristics of mesenteric lymphadenitis?**

Vague, migratory abdominal pain that is usually self-limiting.

❏❏ **What is Fothergill's sign?**

A bluish discoloration of the skin overlying the rectus sheath.

❏❏ **What syndrome is associated with multiple desmoid tumors?**

Gardner's syndrome (familial polyposis coli).

❏❏ **What diagnostic modalities are most useful in identifying rectus sheath hematomas?**

CT and MRI.

☐☐ **T/F: Mesenteric tumors are usually cystic.**

True.

☐☐ **What is the treatment of choice for patients with desmoid tumors?**

Wide surgical excision.

☐☐ **A 28 year old female presents with a palpable abdominal mass, which, upon investigation, reveals an unencapsulated benign hard fibroma. What is the most likely diagnosis?**

A desmoid tumor.

☐☐ **What is the function of the omentum?**

Fixation of the viscera and transmission of the vascular supply.

☐☐ **What is the most common presentation of patients with retroperitoneal fibrosis?**

Dull, non-colicky back, flank or abdominal pain.

☐☐ **What is the diagnostic test of choice for retroperitoneal fibrosis?**

Intravenous pyelography (IVP).

☐☐ **What are the most common causes of pseudocysts of the omentum?**

Fat necrosis, trauma with hematoma or a foreign body reaction.

☐☐ **T/F: Women are more commonly affected by dermoid tumors than men.**

True.

☐☐ **What finding is diagnostic of a dermoid cyst?**

The presence of bone or teeth.

☐☐ **What are the goals of treatment for patients with retroperitoneal fibrosis?**

Identification and management of potential causative agents, relief of ureteral obstruction and reversal of the inflammatory-fibrotic process.

☐☐ **What is the most common solid tumor of the omentum?**

Metastatic carcinoma.

☐☐ **What is the root of the mesentery?**

The ligament of Treitz (duodenojejunal flexure).

☐☐ **What anatomical structure(s) run between the two fused layers of the abdominal peritoneum?**

The intestinal branches of the superior mesenteric artery and vein.

☐☐ **Other than for the transport of nutrients, what is the major function of the mesenteric vascular bed?**

Maintenance of bodily hemostasis.

❑❑ **What percentage of the cardiac output goes to the splanchnic (vascular) bed?**

25 to 30%.

❑❑ **What is the arterial supply to the jejunum and ileum?**

The superior mesenteric artery (SMA).

❑❑ **What are the most common benign tumors of the mesentery?**

Lipomas and fibromas.

❑❑ **What structures are supplied by the inferior mesenteric artery (IMA)?**

The left transverse colon, descending colon, sigmoid colon and the proximal part of the rectum.

❑❑ **What is the most common presenting symptom of acute occlusion of SMA?**

Severe abdominal pain out of proportion to physical findings.

❑❑ **If the diagnosis of acute mesenteric ischemia is considered, what is the proper diagnostic modality?**

Immediate mesenteric angiography.

❑❑ **What is the most common cause of splanchnic artery aneurysms?**

Arteriosclerosis.

❑❑ **What percentage of splanchnic artery aneurysms rupture?**

2 to 10%.

❑❑ **What are the major symptoms of splanchnic aneurysm rupture into the peritoneal cavity?**

Sudden, severe abdominal pain rapidly followed by circulatory collapse.

❑❑ **What is the classic triad seen in patients with hemobilia?**

Gastrointestinal bleeding, biliary colic and jaundice.

❑❑ **What is the definitive study for the diagnosis of splanchnic artery aneurysm?**

Selective mesenteric angiography.

❑❑ **What are the most common malignant tumors of the mesentery?**

Liposarcoma and leiomyosarcoma.

❑❑ **Where in the mesentery do most tumors occur?**

Approximately two-thirds are located in the mesentery of the small intestine, usually that of the ileum.

❑❑ **What is contained within the retroperitoneum?**

The kidneys, ureters, adrenal glands, portions of the intestinal tract, particularly the duodenum, portions of the autonomic nervous system and lymphatics.

❏❏ **What are the most common presenting symptoms of a retroperitoneal tumor?**

An enlarging abdomen, backache, a sense of fullness or heaviness and a vague, indefinite pain that may become severe and radicular.

❏❏ **Why is complete excision of retroperitoneal sarcomas possible in only about 25% of patients?**

Because of their proximity to nonresectable structures.

ADRENAL, PITUITARY AND HYPOTHALAMUS PEARLS

The man who makes no mistakes does not usually make anything.
Edward John Phelps

❏❏ **Primary adrenal insufficiency refers to destruction of which component of the hypothalamus-hypophyseal-adrenal (HPA) axis?**

The adrenal gland.

❏❏ **What is the most common cause of chronic primary adrenal insufficiency (Addison's Disease)?**

Autoimmune disease.

❏❏ **What are the most common causes of acute primary adrenal insufficiency?**

Adrenal hemorrhage, meningococcal disease, sepsis, anticoagulation therapy and the antiphospholipid syndrome.

❏❏ **What diseases may produce a slow, insidious progression to primary adrenal insufficiency?**

Autoimmune diseases, tuberculosis, systemic fungal infections, CMV, Kaposi's sarcoma, metastatic carcinoma and lymphoma.

❏❏ **What are the clinical manifestations of adrenal insufficiency?**

Fatigue, lethargy, anorexia, weight loss, depression, dizziness, orthostatic hypotension, nausea, vomiting, diarrhea, hyponatremia, hyperkalemia, hypoglycemia, normochromic/normocytic anemia, lymphocytosis and eosinophilia.

❏❏ **What tests are used to evaluate secondary adrenal insufficiency?**

The insulin-induced hypoglycemia test, the short metyrapone test and the corticotropin releasing hormone (CRH) test.

❏❏ **T/F: Imaging studies of the adrenal glands are necessary in the evaluation of patients with primary adrenal insufficiency.**

True.

❏❏ **What is the initial daily replacement of hydrocortisone once a patient with adrenal insufficiency is stabilized?**

15 mg in the morning and 10 mg in the evening. The dose should be the smallest possible to alleviate clinical symptoms yet prevent weight gain and osteoporosis.

❏❏ **What general precautions should be taken by all patients with adrenal insufficiency?**

1. They should wear a medic alert bracelet.

2. They should carry a card detailing their medications and recommendations for treatment in emergencies.
3. They should double or triple the dose of hydrocortisone when they sustain significant injury or illness.
4. They should secure ampules of glucocorticoids for self injection or suppositories when vomiting or unable to take anything by mouth.

❏❏ **What accounts for cortisol's almost immediate effect on blood pressure in patients with adrenal insufficiency?**

Cortisol exerts a permissive effect on catecholamine vascular responsivity. It also has a vital role in the maintenance of vascular tone, vascular permeability and the distribution of body water within the vascular compartment.

❏❏ **How much increased cortisol production accompanies surgery?**

It depends upon the surgery; 85% above baseline for up to 2 days post-laparotomy and 35% above baseline for more minor procedures.

❏❏ **What is the relationship between the serum cortisol level and the illness severity score?**

The higher the score, the higher the cortisol level and the higher the mortality.

❏❏ **Which drugs can increase the metabolism of cortisol?**

Phenytoin, phenobarbital and rifampin.

❏❏ **What symptoms should increase the suspicion of adrenal insufficiency in critically ill patients?**

Unexplained circulatory instability, high fever without an identifiable source, nonresponsive to antibiotics, hypoglycemia, hyponatremia, hyperkalemia, neutropenia, eosinophilia, unexplained mental status changes and disparity between the anticipated severity of disease and the actual state of the patient.

❏❏ **What is the normal daily production of cortisol?**

5 mg/m^2.

❏❏ **What are the adverse effects of excessive cortisol dosing for patients in high-stress situations?**

Catabolic effects on muscle, impaired wound healing, inhibition of insulin and anti-inflammatory effects on active infection.

❏❏ **What are the current recommendations for stress doses of cortisol in patients with suspected adrenal insufficiency?**

Minor stress, 25 mg/day, moderate stress; 50 to 75 mg/day and major stress, 100 to 150 mg/day.

❏❏ **What hormones contribute to serum glucose control in uncomplicated starvation?**

Insulin and glucagon.

❏❏ **What is the ebb phase of the metabolic response to stress?**

It occurs just after injury and is characterized by a generalized decrease in metabolism. Cardiac output, metabolic rate and body temperature are all decreased, while sympathetic activity and serum glucose are increased.

❏❏ **T/F: The stress response usually results in hypoglycemia.**

False.

❏❏ **How much cortisol is produced by the adrenal glands in response to the stress of surgery?**

75 to 150 mg/day in response to a major surgery and approximately 50 mg/day after a minor procedure.

❏❏ **What stimulates growth hormone (GH) secretion?**

Growth hormone-releasing hormone (GH-RH)

❏❏ **T/F: GH is decreased during periods of stress.**

False.

❏❏ **What are the stimuli for aldosterone secretion?**

ACTH, angiotensin II, increased serum potassium and decreased serum sodium.

❏❏ **What are the effects of alpha- and beta-adrenergic stimulation on insulin and glucagon secretion?**

Stimulation of alpha-receptors on beta islet cells inhibits insulin secretion while stimulation of the beta-receptors increases insulin release. The alpha islet cells have only beta-receptors which lead to an increase in glucagon release when stimulated.

❏❏ **What is the effect of beta-endorphins during times of injury or stress?**

Hypotension.

❏❏ **What enzymes are involved in the production of angiontensin II from its precursors?**

Renin and angiotensin converting enzyme (ACE).

❏❏ **What hormones stimulate the mobilization of fatty acids from fat stores in the body during periods of stress?**

Catecholamines, cortisol and glucagon.

❏❏ **What is the blood supply to the posterior lobe of the pituitary gland?**

The inferior hypophyseal artery, a branch from the carotid artery.

❏❏ **What is the drainage of the long hypophyseal portal veins?**

The cavernous sinus.

❏❏ **T/F: Women have a larger pituitary gland than men.**

True.

❏❏ **What is the composition of the neurohypophysis?**

The posterior lobe of the pituitary, the pituitary stalk and the median eminence.

❏❏ **Where is the hypophysis (pituitary gland) located?**

Within the sella turcica.

❏❏ **What hormones are synthesized from the supraoptic and paraventricular nuclei?**

Antidiuretic hormone (ADH) and oxytocin.

❏❏ **Just lateral to the sella turcica is the cavernous sinus, which contains what structures?**

The carotid arteries and cranial nerves III, IV and VI.

❏❏ **What forms the roof of the sella turcica?**

The diaphragma sella, a thick reflection of the dura mater.

❏❏ **In what percentage of individuals does the diaphragma sella closely encircle the pituitary stalk, thus, acting as an anatomic barrier?**

50%.

❏❏ **What is the action of oxytocin?**

It stimulates uterine contraction during labor and elicits milk ejection by its action on the myoepithelial cells of the mammary ducts.

❏❏ **What stimulates the release of ACTH?**

Hypothalamic corticotropin-releasing factor (CRF) and circulating glucocorticoids.

❏❏ **What is the action of ADH?**

It causes an increased rate of sodium and chloride reabsorption and it enhances permeability within the collecting ducts of the renal medulla.

❏❏ **What is the function of LH in the adult male?**

It stimulates Leydig cells to produce testosterone.

❏❏ **What is the result of excess secretion of GH prior to closure of the epiphysis of long bones?**

Gigantism.

❏❏ **What is the result of increased cellular levels of cAMP?**

Conversion of cholesterol to androgens, estrogens and corticosteroid precursors as well as synthesis of mineralocorticoids (aldosterone).

❏❏ **Under normal circumstances, when is the plasma ACTH and serum cortisol at its lowest level?**

Between 10:00 P.M. and 2:00 A.M. (The highest level occurs at approximately 8:00 A.M.)

❏❏ **What are the actions of the enkephalins and endorphins?**

They have potent analgesic properties and influence the release of pituitary hormones (i.e., LH, PRL and vasopressin).

❏❏ **What stimulates release of the endogenous opioids?**

Periods of stress, shock or hypoglycemia.

❏❏ **What are the effects of GH?**

1. It elicits longitudinal growth of the skeleton.
2. It antagonizes the effects of insulin in peripheral tissues.
3. It stimulates insulin secretion from the pancreas.
4. It directly stimulates liver cell growth and adipocyte metabolism.
5. It increases the serum levels of free fatty acids.

❑❑ **Where are somatomedins synthesized?**

In the liver.

❑❑ **What stimulates the release of GH?**

Stress, exercise, hypoglycemia, protein depletion and administration of glucagon and L-dopa.

❑❑ **What cells within the pituitary secrete prolactin?**

Lactotrophs.

❑❑ **What is the function of prolactin?**

It initiates and sustains lactation by the breast glands. It may also influence synthesis and release of progesterone by the ovary and testosterone by the testis.

❑❑ **What is the imaging modality of choice when a pituitary lesion is suspected?**

MRI.

❑❑ **What is renal diabetes insipidis?**

Failure of the kidneys to respond to an elevation of serum vasopressin.

❑❑ **What is Sheehan's syndrome?**

Postpartum infarction and necrosis of the pituitary.

❑❑ **T/F: Cushing's disease is more common in men.**

False. It is 8 times more common in women.

❑❑ **Excess GH secretion produces what clinical syndrome in adults?**

Acromegaly.

❑❑ **What is the best surgical approach to the pituitary?**

The transnasal transsphenoidal approach.

❑❑ **What is the syndrome of inappropriate antidiuretic hormone (SIADH)?**

Hypersecretion of vasopressin.

❑❑ **What is the drainage of the left adrenal vein?**

The left renal vein.

❑❑ **What is the precursor for all adrenal steroids?**

Cholesterol.

❏❏ **What conditions increase the level of plasma cortisol binding globulin (CBG)?**

Pregnancy, estrogen supplements, oral contraceptives and hyperthyroidism.

❏❏ **What is the physiologically active form of plasma cortisol?**

Free cortisol.

❏❏ **What physiologic stimuli cause the adrenal gland to secrete cortisol?**

A decrease in blood volume, tissue damage, hypoxia, deviations in body temperature and hypoglycemia.

❏❏ **What tissues/organs are glucose independent?**

The liver, brain and erythrocytes.

❏❏ **What are the metabolic effects of glucocorticoids?**

1. It stimulates release of glucose from peripheral tissues.
2. It stimulates liver gluconeogenesis and glycogen deposition.
3. It inhibits protein synthesis in peripheral tissues.
4. It stimulates degradation of proteins in peripheral tissues.
5. It stimulates protein synthesis in the liver.

❏❏ **T/F: The net metabolic effect of glucocorticoids include hyperglycemia, a negative nitrogen balance and lipogenesis.**

False.

❏❏ **What are the effects of glucocorticoids on the immune system?**

1. They block interleukins, leukotrienes, histamine and bradykinin.
2. They inhibit the release of arachidonic acid and thromboxane.
3. They inhibit the local increase in vascular permeability caused by serotonin.
4. They inhibit macrophage and neutrophil chemotaxis.
5. They decrease the serum complement level.
6. They suppress natural killer cell activity.

❏❏ **What is the precursor in aldosterone synthesis?**

Progesterone.

❏❏ **Where is aldosterone produced?**

In the zona glomerulosa of the adrenal cortex.

❏❏ **What physiologic stimuli causes release of aldosterone?**

A decrease in the circulating blood volume and an increase in the serum potassium concentration.

❏❏ **Where is aldosterone primarily metabolized?**

The liver.

❏❏ **What physiologic stimuli cause secretion of renin?**

A decrease in the arterial pressure in the renal afferent arteries, a decrease in chloride concentration in the renal tubules and stimulation of the renal sympathetic nerves.

❏❏ **What cells secrete renin?**

The juxtaglomerular cells of the kidney.

❏❏ **What is the function of renin?**

It cleaves angiotensinogin to form angiotensin I.

❏❏ **What is the function of angiotensin II?**

It is a potent vasoconstrictor that plays an important role in blood pressure maintenance.

❏❏ **What is the most common cause of Cushing's syndrome?**

A pituitary microadenoma.

❏❏ **What tumor most commonly causes ectopic ACTH secretion?**

Small-cell carcinoma of the lung.

❏❏ **What is the most common tumor of the pituitary gland?**

A chromophobe adenoma.

❏❏ **What is the expected result of the dexamethasone suppression test in a patient with an ectopic source of ACTH secretion?**

Dexamthasone should fail to suppress cortisol secretion.

❏❏ **What enzyme converts angiotensin I to angiotensin II?**

Angiotensin converting enzyme (in the lung).

❏❏ **T/F: Virilizing adrenal tumors are more common in females than in males.**

True. They are twice as common in females.

❏❏ **What tests are useful in differentiating hypercortisolism due to pituitary sources of ACTH from those due to ectopic sources of ACTH?**

The dexamethasone suppression test and the metyrapone test.

❏❏ **What is the most common cause of primary hyperaldosteronism?**

A solitary adrenal adenoma.

❏❏ **What enzymatic deficiency is associated with most cases of the adrenogenital syndrome (congenital adrenal hyperplasia)?**

21-hydroxylase.

❏❏ **What is the major catecholamine produced in the adrenal medulla?**

Epinephrine.

❏❏ **What is the rate-limiting step in catecholamine synthesis?**

Hydroxylation of tyrosine to dihydroxy-phenylalanine (DOPA) by tyrosine hydroxylase.

❏❏ **What is the etiology of Nelson's syndrome?**

Continued growth of ACTH-secreting pituitary microadenomas.

❏❏ **What is Waterhouse-Freiderichsen syndrome?**

Acute adrenal hemorrhage secondary to sepsis.

❏❏ **What is the only chemotherapeutic agent that has been proven to be of some value in the treatment of adrenal carcinoma?**

Mitotane.

❏❏ **What is the most common cause of acute adrenocortical insufficiency?**

Withdrawal of chronic steroid therapy.

❏❏ **What is the most common cause of spontaneous adrenal insufficiency?**

Autoimmune destruction of the adrenal glands (greater than 80%).

❏❏ **What are the classic signs of adrenal crisis?**

Hypotension, hypoglycemia and hyperkalemia.

❏❏ **What is the most useful test to evaluate a patient suspected of having adrenocortical insufficiency?**

The rapid ACTH stimulation test.

❏❏ **What is the appropriate management for patients with acute adrenocortical insufficiency?**

Hydrocortisone (100 mg every 6 hours for 24 hours), correction of volume depletion, dehydration, hypotension and hypoglycemia and correction of precipitating factors.

❏❏ **What are the classic clinical manifestations of primary hyperaldosteronism?**

Hypertension with spontaneous hypokalemia.

❏❏ **What is the biochemical test of choice to differentiate between hyperplasia and adenoma as the cause of primary hyperaldosteronism?**

Measurement of plasma aldosterone concentration after a change in posture. Only patients with an adenoma experience a postural decrease in aldosterone.

❏❏ **What is the best noninvasive test to localize an aldosteronoma?**

CT scan.

❏❏ **What is the effect of a C-21 deficiency in females? In males?**

It causes pseudohermaphrodites in females and macrogenitosomia praecox (enlarged external genitalia) in males.

❏❏ **What is the etiology of congenital adrenogenital hyperplasia (CAH)?**

Adrenal androgen hypersecretion.

❐❐ **What is the classic symptom of androgen excess?**

Hirsutism.

❐❐ **What is the treatment for patients with CAH?**

Glucocorticoid administration to suppress ACTH.

❐❐ **What test rules out CAH?**

Failure of the dexamethasone suppression test.

❐❐ **What hormones are synthesized and secreted by the adrenal medulla?**

Epinephrine, norepinephrine and small amounts of dopamine.

❐❐ **What is the precursor for all catecholamines?**

Tyrosine.

❐❐ **What are the major enzymes that metabolize catecholamines?**

Monoamineoxidase (MAO) and catechol-o-methyl transferase (COMT).

❐❐ **Pheochromocytomas are tumors derived from what cells?**

Chromaffin cells.

❐❐ **What percentage of pheochromocytomas are malignant?**

10%. (Remember the rules of 10s pheochromocytomas.)

❐❐ **What percentage of neuroblastomas are intraadrenal?**

40 to 50%.

❐❐ **What is the most common presentation of a patient with a neuroblastoma?**

An asymptomatic patient with an irregular, firm intraabdominal mass.

❐❐ **What is the incidence of neuroblastomas in children?**

Neuroblastomas represent 7% of all childhood cancers. It is the third most common malignancy in childhood (behind brain tumors and hematopoetic-reticular endothelial cell malignancies).

❐❐ **What are the most common locations of a neuroblastoma?**

Intraabdominal and retroperitoneal (60 to 70%).

❐❐ **What are the characteristic signs of adrenal insufficiency?**

Hyperkalemia and hyperpigmentation.

❐❐ **What syndromes are associated with pheochromocytomas?**

MEN-IIa, MEN-IIb, von Recklinghausen's disease, tuberous sclerosis and Sturge-Weber disease.

❑❑ **What hormones are secreted by the anterior pituitary?**

GH, ACTH, TSH, LH, FSH and prolactin.

THYROID AND PARATHYROID PEARLS

Little minds are interested in the extraordinary; great minds in the commonplace.
Elbert Hubbard

❏❏ **What is the principle secretory product of the thyroid gland?**

Thyroxine (T4).

❏❏ **What is the arterial blood supply to the thyroid gland?**

The paired superior thyroid and inferior thyroid arteries and, occasionally, the thyroid ima artery.

❏❏ **What is the venous drainage of the thyroid gland?**

The superior and middle thyroid veins drain into the internal jugular vein and the inferior thyroid veins drain into the innominate vein.

❏❏ **What hormone regulates iodine uptake and oxidation?**

Thyroid stimulating hormone (TSH).

❏❏ **What is the principle metabolically active thyroid hormone?**

Triiodothyronine (T3).

❏❏ **Removal of the inner iodine ring of T4 by deiodination produces which form of thyroid hormone?**

Reverse T3 (rT3).

❏❏ **What is the function of rT3?**

It is biologically inactive.

❏❏ **What is the major thyroid hormone-binding protein?**

Thyronine binding globulin (TBG).

❏❏ **T/F: Laboratory measurements of thyroid hormone include bound hormone.**

True.

❏❏ **What factors increase TSH secretion?**

Iodide, lithium and radiocontrast agents. (Minor increases are seen with dopamine antagonists, chlorpromazine, cimetidine, haloperidol and metoclopromide.)

❏❏ **What is the most common type of thyroid carcinoma?**

Papillary.

❏❏ **What type of thyroid carcinoma has the best prognosis?**

Papillary.

❏❏ **T/F: Changes in the amount or affinity of the binding proteins can have major effects on total serum levels.**

True.

❏❏ **What is the free T4 index (FTI)?**

FTI = Total T4 x T3 resin uptake.

❏❏ **T/F: FTI is increased in hypothyroidism.**

False.

❏❏ **T/F: Patients with documented euthyroid sick syndrome are treated with supplemental thyroid hormone.**

False.

❏❏ **What autoantibodies are associated with Grave's disease?**

Long-acting thyroid stimulator (LATS) and thyroid-stimulating immunoglobulin (TSI).

❏❏ **What are the signs and symptoms of hyperthyroidism?**

Anxiety, weight loss, heat intolerance, gastrointestinal disturbances, fever, muscle weakness and tremors.

❏❏ **What is the differential diagnosis of thyrotoxicosis?**

Sepsis, pheochromocytoma, cocaine/amphetamine overdose, neuroleptic malignant syndrome and malignant hyperthermia.

❏❏ **What is the first thyroid function test abnormality seen in patients with hypothyroidism?**

TSH elevation (usually associated with a low T4).

❏❏ **T/F: Thyroid function tests must be done prior to the initiation of treatment for thyroid storm.**

False.

❏❏ **What type of thyroiditis is associated with retroperitoneal fibrosis?**

Riedel's thyroiditis.

❏❏ **What is the function of TSH?**

It increases the rate of iodide transport, thyroglobulin synthesis, T3 and T4 formation and release and it increases the size and vascularity of the thyroid gland (trophic effect).

❏❏ **What laboratory values suggest a central cause of hypothyroidism?**

A low serum T4 in the presence of an inappropriately low TSH level.

❑❑ **What is the anatomic relationship of the recurrent laryngeal nerve to the posteromedial suspensory ligament of the thyroid (ligament of Berry)?**

The recurrent laryngeal nerve usually lies just lateral to this ligament, closely approximated to the thyroid lobe. However, it runs into the ligament in 25% of patients. This is the most common site of injury to the nerve.

❑❑ **What is the result of bilateral recurrent laryngeal nerve injury?**

Paralysis of the vocal cords with resultant airway compromise.

❑❑ **What is the result of unilateral injury to the superior laryngeal nerve?**

Inability to forcefully project one's voice or sing high notes.

❑❑ **T/F: Papillary thyroid carcinoma has a high propensity for multicentricity.**

True.

❑❑ **What is the mechanism of action of propylthiouracil (PTU)?**

PTU interferes with the incorporation of iodine into the tyrosine residues of thyroglobulin, preventing oxidation of iodide to iodine. It also inhibits the peripheral conversion of T4 to T3.

❑❑ **What test is diagnostic for Grave's disease?**

Diffuse, increased uptake of 131I within a symmetrically enlarged gland.

❑❑ **A 35 year old female presents with a diffuse, slowly growing goiter, weight gain, fatigue and cold intolerance. What is the most likely diagnosis?**

Hashimoto's thyroiditis.

❑❑ **What is the indication for performing a radionuclide scan for a patient with a solitary thyroid nodule?**

Evidence of hyperthyroidism.

❑❑ **What is the single most important test in the diagnostic work-up of a patient with a solitary thyroid nodule?**

Fine needle aspiration (FNA).

❑❑ **A 46 year old female with no clinical risk factors presents with a palpable thyroid nodule. Fluid is returned on FNA, the nodule disappeared and the cytology is benign. What is the next step in management?**

Follow-up. The cyst may recur, requiring repeat aspiration.

❑❑ **T/F: Nodal metastases are more common than distant metastases in patients with follicular thyroid carcinoma.**

False.

❑❑ **A 45 year old male with no risk factors presents with a thyroid nodule. Fluid is returned on FNA, the nodule shrink but does not completely disappear and the cytology is benign. What is the treatment of choice?**

Total thyroid lobectomy and isthmusectomy.

❑❑ **A 62 year old female presents with a thyroid nodule, no risk factors and a non-diagnostic FNA. What is the treatment of choice?**

Total thyroid lobectomy and isthmusectomy.

❑❑ **What is minimal papillary thyroid carcinoma?**

A papillary carcinoma less than 1 cm in size with no clinically evident lymph node involvement.

❑❑ **What factor best correlates with the presence of lymph note metastases in papillary carcinoma?**

Age.

❑❑ **What variants of papillary thyroid carcinoma are associated with a worse prognosis?**

Insular, columnar and tall cell variants.

❑❑ **T/F: The PTH level is inversely related to the serum calcium level.**

True.

❑❑ **Follicular carcinoma metastases occur primarily by what route?**

Hematogenous dissemination to the lungs, bones and other peripheral tissues.

❑❑ **What is the treatment of choice for patients with follicular thyroid carcinoma?**

Total lobectomy and isthmusectomy.

❑❑ **What is the surgical treatment for patients with medullary thyroid carcinoma (MTC)?**

Total thyroidectomy with central node dissection, lateral cervical lymph node sampling of palpable nodes and a modified radical neck dissection if positive.

❑❑ **Which thyroid carcinomas respond to radioactive iodine?**

Papillary and follicular carcinomas.

❑❑ **What is the order of frequency for phenotypic presentation of the abnormalities seen in MEN 2A?**

Medullary thyroid carcinoma (100%), pheochromocytoma (40%) and parathyroid hyperplasia (20% to 30%).

❑❑ **What are the components of the MEN-2B syndrome?**

Medullary thyroid carcinoma, pheochromocytoma, mucosal neuromas, ganglioneuromas and a marfanoid habitus.

❑❑ **What laboratory values should be obtained prior to operative management for a patient with MTC?**

PTH, serum calcium and urinary metanephrine and vanillylmandelic acid (VMA) levels.

❑❑ **What cells secrete calcitonin?**

The parafollicular (C-cells) within the thyroid gland.

❑❑ **What is the embryologic etiology of the parathyroid glands?**

The inferior parathyroid glands originate from the third pharyngeal pouch and the superior thyroid glands originate from the fourth pharyngeal pouch.

❑❑ **What percentage of individuals have more than 4 parathyroids?**

Up to 15%.

❑❑ **Which organs are directly affected by PTH?**

Bone and kidney.

❑❑ **Which organs are affected by vitamin D?**

Intestines and bone.

❑❑ **How is the active form of vitamin D (calcitriol) synthesized?**

In the skin, previtamin D3 (activated 7-dehydrocholesterol) is synthesized photochemically from 7-dehydrocholesterol and is slowly isomerized to vitamin D3. Vitamin D3 is converted in the liver to 25-(OH)D3, the major circulating form. It undergoes enterohepatic circulation and is reabsorbed from the gut. In the kidney, it is further hydroxylated to the much more metabolically active form $1,25\text{-}(OH_2)D3$ (calcitriol).

❑❑ **T/F: The inferior parathyroid glands are more likely to be ectopically located than the superior glands.**

True.

❑❑ **What is the differential diagnosis of hypercalcemia?**

Hyperparathyroidism, malignancy, vitamin A or D intoxication, thiazide diuretics, hyperthyroidism, milk-alkali syndrome, sarcoidosis, familiar hypocalciuric, hypercalcemic hyperparathyroidism, immobilization, Paget's disease, lithium, Addisonian crisis and idiopathic hypercalcemia of infancy.

❑❑ **What chloride/phosphate ratio is highly suggestive of hyperparathyroidism?**

Greater than 30.

❑❑ **What osseous characteristic is pathognomonic for hyperparathyroidism?**

Osteitis fibrosa cystica.

❑❑ **What is the etiology of familial hypocalciuric, hypercalcemic hyperparathyroidism?**

A defect in the calcium-sensing receptor.

❑❑ **What clinical characteristics are associated with primary hyperparathyroidism?**

Urolithiasis, hypercalciuria, emotional disorders, osteoporosis, diminished renal function, hyperparathyroid bone disease and peptic ulcer disease.

❑❑ **What percentage of patients with primary hyperparathyroidism have a single adenoma?**

80%.

❐❐ **What localization studies should be performed before parathyroid exploration for patients with primary hyperparathyroidism?**

Typically none. In the hands of an experienced surgeon, the cure rate for primary hyperparathyroidism at the initial operation, without localization studies, exceeds 95%.

❐❐ **What are the characteristics of parathyroid carcinoma?**

A palpable neck mass, a serum calcium greater than 14 mg/dl and unusually severe symptoms. Patients often have elevated levels of human chorionic gonadotropin (HCG).

❐❐ **What is persistent hyperparathyroidism?**

Continued elevation of serum calcium levels postoperatively or its development within 6 months of operation.

❐❐ **What is the most common cause of persistent hyperparathyroidism?**

A missed hyperfunctioning parathyroid gland.

❐❐ **What is recurrent hyperparathyroidism?**

Development of elevated serum calcium levels more than 6 months after operation.

❐❐ **What are the indications for surgical therapy for patients with secondary hyperparathyroidism?**

Medical intractability, bone pain, pathologic fractures, ectopic calcification and intractable pruritus.

❐❐ **What is most common cause of hypoparathyroidism?**

Thyroid surgery.

❐❐ **What is the first line therapy for patients with marked hypercalcemia and/or severe symptoms?**

Intravenous hydration followed by furosemide.

❐❐ **What are the indications for calcium supplementation after thyroid or parathyroid surgery?**

Circumoral paresthesias, anxiety, positive Chvostek's or Trousseau's sign, tetany, ECG changes or serum calcium less than 7.1 ml/dl.

❐❐ **What is the immediate treatment for patients with acute symptomatic hypocalcemia?**

Intravenous calcium gluconate.

TRAUMA AND BURN PEARLS

If you are too smart to pay the doctor, you had better be too smart to get ill.
African proverb

□□ **What is the most sensitive indicator of shock in children?**

Tachycardia.

□□ **What initial fluid bolus should be given to children in shock?**

20 ml/kg.

□□ **What topical antimicrobial agent is associated with neutropenia and thrombocytopenia?**

Silver sulfadiazine.

□□ **When does a subdural hematoma become isodense?**

1 to 3 weeks post-bleed.

□□ **What percentage of cervical spine fractures in adults are identifiable on lateral x-rays?**

90%.

□□ **What are the absolute indications for neck exploration following penetrating trauma?**

Persistent hemorrhage, pulsatile hematoma, coma, stroke, crepitance, dysphonia, palpable laryngeal injury, stridor, hemoptysis, hematemesis and odynophagia.

□□ **What is the daily calorie requirement for a 75 kg male with a 20% TBSA burn?**

2,675 Kcal (25 Kcal/kg + 40 Kcal per percent TBSA burn).

□□ **What is the treatment of choice for patients with a tension pneumothorax?**

Needle decompression at the second intercostal space, in the midclavicular line.

□□ **What is the most common source of intrathoracic bleeding?**

The lungs.

□□ **What is the most important cause of hypoxia in a patient with a flail chest?**

The underlying lung contusion.

□□ **What is Hamman's sign?**

A crunching sound heard over the heart during systole secondary to pneumomediastinum.

□□ **What is the most common complaint in a patient with a traumatic aortic injury?**

Retrosternal or intrascapular pain.

❐❐ **What minimal blood pressure is indicated by a palpable radial pulse?**

80 mm Hg.

❐❐ **What are the absolute indications for invasive airway management?**

Obstruction, apnea, hypoxia and severe neck trauma.

❐❐ **Which long bone is most commonly fractured?**

The tibia.

❐❐ **What is included in the differential diagnosis of distended neck veins in a trauma patient?**

Tension pneumothorax, pericardial tamponade, air embolism and cardiac failure.

❐❐ **What are the compartments of the leg?**

Anterior, lateral, deep posterior and superficial posterior.

❐❐ **A 40 year old male unrestrained driver in a high-speed motor vehicle crash (MVA) presents with multiple rib fractures and is in respiratory distress with paradoxical chest motion. What is the most likely diagnosis?**

A flail chest.

❐❐ **What rib fracture has the worst prognosis?**

The first rib.

❐❐ **What signs and symptoms are associated with compartment syndrome involving the deep posterior compartment of the leg?**

Pain on foot eversion or toe dorsiflexion and hypesthesia of the plantar surface of the foot.

❐❐ **What compartment pressure mandates fasciotomy?**

Greater than 30 mm Hg.

❐❐ **What are the major wounding mechanisms of ballistic injuries?**

Tissue crush and stretch.

❐❐ **What cardiovascular injury is commonly associated with sternal fractures?**

Blunt myocardial injury.

❐❐ **How much fluid in the chest cavity is required to be visible on a decubitus or upright chest x-rays?**

200 to 300 ml.

❐❐ **What is Beck's triad?**

Muffled heart tones, hypotension and distended neck veins seen with pericardial tamponade.

○○ **What valve is most commonly injured in blunt trauma?**

The aortic valve.

○○ **What are the basic mechanisms for elevated compartment pressure?**

External compression and volume increase within the compartment.

○○ **What anatomic locations of bullets/pellets are associated with lead intoxication?**

Within the bursa, joints and disc spaces.

○○ **Which fractures are most frequently associated with compartment syndrome?**

Tibia and supracondylar humerus fractures.

○○ **Why are civilian bullets usually more damaging than military bullets?**

Military bullets are usually jacketed and are less prone to fragmentation/mushrooming than hollow/soft point civilian bullets.

○○ **What tissues are more prone to significant wounding secondary to temporary cavitation?**

Less elastic tissues (e.g., brain, spleen and liver), fluid-filled organs (e.g., bladder, bowel and heart) and dense tissue (e.g., bone).

○○ **Why do simple through-and-through wounds of the extremities fare well regardless of the velocity of the bullet?**

The short path in the tissue results in little or no deformation of slower bullets and less time for the higher velocity bullet to yaw.

○○ **T/F: The heat of firing is significant enough to sterilize a bullet and its wound.**

False. Contaminants from the body surface and viscera can be carried along the bullet's path.

○○ **What method of airway control is indicated in a patient with severe maxillofacial trauma?**

Cricothyroidotomy.

○○ **What anatomical features of the brain and skull influence the severity of head wounds?**

The brain has minimal elasticity or cohesiveness. Thus, it is highly sensitive to cavitation. In addition, the calvarium is immobile in adults and contains the cavitation forces.

○○ **Other than lead intoxication, why should intraarticular bullets be removed?**

They may lead to synovitis and severe damage to the articular cartilage.

○○ **What organ is most frequently injured in blunt trauma?**

Spleen.

○○ **What is Kehr's sign?**

Left shoulder pain with splenic rupture.

❑❑ **What is the most common cause of early death after myocardial contusion?**

Arrhythmias (usually within the first 6 hours).

❑❑ **What is the most common site of a basilar skull fracture?**

The petrous portion of the temporal bone.

❑❑ **What artery is the most commonly associated with development of an epidural hematoma?**

The middle meningeal artery.

❑❑ **What is the diagnostic test of choice for evaluation of retroperitoneal organs in trauma patients?**

CT scan.

❑❑ **What are the most unstable cervical spine injuries?**

A transverse atlantal ligament rupture, a dens fracture and burst fractures with posterior ligament disruption.

❑❑ **What is the best measure of adequate burn resuscitation?**

Urine output.

❑❑ **What is the Cushing reflex?**

Bradycardia and hypertension associated with brainstem herniation.

❑❑ **What is a Jefferson fracture?**

A burst fracture of the ring of C1.

❑❑ **A 36 year old intoxicated male presents with multiple contusions and lacerations. What is the appropriate method of abdominal evaluation?**

CT scan or diagnostic peritoneal lavage (DPL). (Physical examination is unreliable in a patient with altered mental status.)

❑❑ **What bacterial load is required to cause a wound infection when a foreign body is present?**

100 organisms/per gram of tissue.

❑❑ **What are the boundaries of zone I of the neck?**

From the clavicle to the cricoid cartilage.

❑❑ **What factors decrease the pain associated with local anesthetic administration?**

Buffering the solution with sodium bicarbonate, decreasing the speed of injection and use of a subdermal injection.

❑❑ **What are the hard signs of arterial injury?**

Hemorrhage, distal pulse deficit, expanding or pulsatile hematoma, distal ischemia, bruits and thrills.

❑❑ **Which Salter fracture has the worst prognosis?**

Type V.

❑❑ **What life-threatening complication is most commonly associated with pelvic fractures?**

Severe hemorrhage.

❑❑ **What is the effect of prophylactic antibiotics on burn wound sepsis?**

They promote selection of antibiotic-resistant bacteria.

❑❑ **Why is epinephrine added to local anesthesia?**

To increase the duration of the anesthesia, induce vasoconstriction and decrease bleeding.

❑❑ **What local anesthetic is responsible for most allergic reactions?**

Procaine.

❑❑ **What is the appropriate surgical approach for repair of renal injuries?**

A midline abdominal incision.

❑❑ **What are the 4 C's in determining muscle viability?**

Color, consistency, contraction and circulation.

❑❑ **What is a Hangman's fracture?**

A C2 bilateral pedicle fracture.

❑❑ **What is the most common bacterium seen in cat bite wounds?**

Pasteurella multocida.

❑❑ **T/F: Staples have greater resistance to infection than sutures.**

True.

❑❑ **What types of wounds result in the majority of tetanus cases?**

Lacerations, punctures and crush injuries.

❑❑ **T/F: It is acceptable to clip or shave an eyebrow if needed, to repair the skin.**

False.

❑❑ **Avascular necrosis of the femoral head is associated with a fracture of what area of the femur?**

The neck.

❑❑ **What is the first step in treating a patient with a long bone fracture in which distal pulses are absent?**

Gentle reduction.

❑❑ **What test reliably evaluates the viability of a fetus in a pregnant trauma patient?**

Amniotic fluid analysis.

☐☐ **What steps are involved in evaluating an extremity after traumatic insult?**

Assessment of the circulation followed by neurologic function, bony deformities and soft tissue defects.

☐☐ **How is pain with motion of an extremity, without apparent fracture, best evaluated?**

With motion or stress x-rays.

☐☐ **What is the appropriate method of evaluating the motor function of the radial nerve?**

Thumb extension and abduction.

☐☐ **What complications are associated with delayed treatment of a septal hematoma?**

Aseptic necrosis and septal perforation.

☐☐ **What must be considered in repair of lacerations of the cheek?**

Avoid injury to the facial nerve, parotid duct and/or parotid gland.

☐☐ **What are the clinical hallmarks of compartment syndrome?**

A tense extremity with pain on passive motion and intact distal pulses.

☐☐ **What type of deformity results from improperly treated auricular hematomas?**

A cauliflower ear.

☐☐ **What is a class II splenic injury?**

A laceration that does not extend into the hilum.

☐☐ **T/F: Fractures associated with open wounds should always be explored surgically.**

True.

☐☐ **What is the maximum time limit for salvaging an ischemic limb?**

6 hours.

☐☐ **T/F: When a posterior dislocation of the knee is reduced and a normal vascular examination is obtained, one may be assured that no vascular injury is present.**

False.

☐☐ **What are the treatment modalities used to minimize the risk of infection in a patient with an open fracture?**

Antibiotic therapy, aggressive surgical debridement, fracture stabilization and meticulous wound care.

☐☐ **What is the proper approach for an emergent thoracotomy for a suspected life-threatening cardiac tamponade?**

A left anterolateral thoracotomy.

☐☐ **T/F: A pulmonary contusion is usually noted on the initial chest x-ray after blunt trauma to the chest.**

True.

❏❏ T/F: The initial management for a patient with a sucking chest wound is tube thoracostomy through the wound.

False.

❏❏ What variables comprise the grading system for the Mangled Extremity Syndrome Index (M.E.S.I.)?

The injury severity score (ISS), integument, nerves, vascular structures, bony structures, lag time, age, pre-existing disease and shock.

❏❏ What type of bodily tissue offers the most resistance to current flow?

Bone.

❏❏ What is the hallmark of electrical injuries?

Extensive deep tissue damage that is far out of proportion to the visible cutaneous burn.

❏❏ What are the immediate priorities in the management of patients with chest trauma?

Secure a stable airway, adequate ventilation and treatment of shock.

❏❏ T/F: Only 10 to 15% of patients with blunt or penetrating trauma to the chest require a formal thoracotomy.

True.

❏❏ What is the most common chronic condition in patients with a chest injury that requires surgical intervention?

Clotted hemothorax.

❏❏ When do irreversible changes to muscles occur following traumatic ischemia?

After 6 hours.

❏❏ The axillary artery is involved in what percentage of extremity vascular trauma?

Less than 10%.

❏❏ What is the most likely diagnosis in a patient with chronic breakdown of a healed burn wound scar?

A Marjolin's ulcer.

❏❏ T/F: Pulse deficit is a reliable sign of axillary artery injury.

False.

❏❏ What type of conduit is preferred for repair of injured vessels?

Autogenous vein grafts.

❏❏ What are the absolute indications for exploration of extremity stab wounds?

Arterial bleeding, limb ischemia and nerve deficit.

❏❏ **The majority of neurologic deficits associated with penetrating trauma to the brachial artery involves which nerve?**

The median nerve.

❏❏ **What is the Pringle maneuver?**

Occlusion of the portal triad.

❏❏ **Which joint dislocation is associated with the highest rate of arterial injuries?**

The knee.

❏❏ **What is the most commonly injured vein?**

The superficial femoral vein.

❏❏ **What is the Fallen Lung Sign?**

A chest x-ray that shows collapse of the lung toward the lateral chest wall.

❏❏ **What is the usual location of a diaphragmatic tear in patients with blunt trauma?**

In the posterolateral region.

❏❏ **T/F: In a patient with persistent or recurrent hypotension and a widened mediastinum on chest x-ray, aortic rupture is the most likely cause of ongoing hemorrhage.**

False.

❏❏ **What is the diagnostic procedure of choice for imaging a suspected great vessel injury?**

Angiography.

❏❏ **What is the most common approach for treatment of compartment syndrome of the lower leg?**

A 2-incision, 4-compartment fasciotomy.

❏❏ **What is the sensory innervation to the nipple?**

T4.

❏❏ **What are the most common indications for extremity fasciotomy?**

1. Greater than 6 hours of limb ischemia.
2. Compartment syndrome.
3. Crush injury.
4. Massive preoperative edema.
5. Combined arterial and venous injuries.
6. Performance of a major venous ligation in the popliteal or femoral area.

❏❏ **Humeral shaft fractures are associated with injury to which upper extremity nerve?**

The radial nerve.

❏❏ **What part of the mandible is most frequently fractured?**

Mandibular fractures occur equally at the condylar-subcondylar area, the angle and in the body-symphysis area (33% each).

☐☐ **T/F: Neural injuries associated with fractures have a greater than 80% chance of spontaneous recovery.**

True.

☐☐ **T/F: Every attempt should be made to salvage the mangled extremity.**

False.

☐☐ **What are the characteristics of the fat embolism syndrome?**

Respiratory insufficiency, mental status changes, thrombocytopenia and petechiae.

☐☐ **Thoracic trauma directly accounts for what percentage of trauma deaths?**

20 to 25%.

☐☐ **What is the most common cause of immediate death following thoracic injury?**

Major disruption of the heart, ascending aorta or descending aorta.

☐☐ **Early death following thoracic injury is usually due to what processes?**

Cardiac tamponade, airway obstruction or uncontrolled hemorrhage.

☐☐ **What percentage of patients with blunt thoracic trauma have a concomitant extrathoracic injury?**

Greater than 75%.

☐☐ **What is the treatment of choice for a patient with a thoracic esophageal injury diagnosed more than 24 hours after injury?**

Wide drainage, esophageal diversion, hyperalimentation and antibiotics.

☐☐ **What associated injury most commonly accompanies blunt chest trauma and requires admission to the hospital?**

A closed head injury.

☐☐ **What artery has a variable origin off the aorta and is implicated in paraplegia with respect to repair of the thoracic aorta?**

The artery of Adamkiewicz.

☐☐ **T/F: A mechanically ventilated patient suspected of having sustained barotrauma must also have a concomitant pneumothorax.**

False.

☐☐ **What is the appropriate management for a large sucking chest wound?**

A flutter-valve dressing.

☐☐ **T/F: A milky white pleural effusion is always a chylothorax.**

False.

❏❏ **What is the initial treatment for a patient with a chylothorax?**

Chest drainage and reduction of enteral fat absorption with bowel rest or medium chain triglycerides (MCT).

❏❏ **Which type of pelvic fracture is most frequently associated with bladder rupture?**

Lateral compression fractures.

❏❏ **How much blood must collect within the pericardial space to produce clinical signs of tamponade?**

As little as 60 to 100 cc.

❏❏ **How much blood return from a chest tube indicates the need for thoracotomy?**

Greater than 1500 ml upon insertion of the chest tube or ongoing bleeding in excess of 200 ml/hr for 4 hours.

❏❏ **What is the treatment of choice for skin that has come into contact with phenol?**

Irrigation with a 50% solution of polyethylene glycol followed by copious water irrigation.

❏❏ **Why are alkaline burns usually more invasive than acid burns?**

Alkaline burns cause damage by liquefaction necrosis. Thus, a barrier of coagulated protein does not form.

❏❏ **What are physical signs of traumatic asphyxia?**

Facial edema, craniocervical cyanosis, petechiae and subconjunctival hemorrhage.

❏❏ **T/F: Stab wounds to zone II of the neck require exploration if they penetrate the platysma.**

True.

❏❏ **What are the indications for observation of patients with penetrating chest wall injuries?**

Stable vital signs, normal bilateral breath sounds and a normal initial chest x-ray.

❏❏ **Which type of current produces the most serious electrical burn injuries?**

Alternating current.

❏❏ **What are the 4 mechanisms by which electricity causes injury?**

Direct contact, conduction, arc and secondary ignition.

❏❏ **At what frequency of alternating current are cardiac arrest and coma most likely to occur?**

50 to 60 cycles/sec.

❏❏ **What is the definition of a high-tension electrical injury?**

Tissue damage caused by greater than 1000 volts.

❏❏ **How is the diagnosis of burn wound sepsis confirmed?**

Presence of greater than 100,000 organism/gram of tissue.

❏❏ **What percentage of burns in children, admitted to hospitals, are intentionally inflicted?**

10%.

❏❏ **How is the common bile duct evaluated intraoperatively with respect to hepatic trauma?**

Cholangiography.

❏❏ **What is the immediate treatment for patients with chemical burns?**

Copious water irrigation.

❏❏ **What is the most important factor in determining the amount of secondary contraction of skin grafts?**

The percentage of dermis in the graft.

❏❏ **What is the mechanism of injury in aortic transection?**

Sudden deceleration (i.e., MVA) which leads to the development of shear forces between the mobile aortic arch and the fixed descending aorta.

❏❏ **What is the current standard for treatment of patients with deep hand burns?**

Early tangential excision and grafting, proper splinting and early mobilization.

❏❏ **What is the most common deformity after a burn injury of the hand?**

Burn syndactyly.

ORTHOPEDIC AND HAND SURGERY PEARLS

Caution: Cape does not enable user to fly.
Batman costume warning label

❑❑ **What serum proteins influence bone induction?**

Platelet-derived growth factor (PDGF), transforming growth factor-beta (TGF-beta), osteogenin and fibroblast growth factor (FGF).

❑❑ **What muscles make up the rotator cuff?**

The teres minor, infraspinatus, supraspinatus and subscapularis.

❑❑ **What is the most frequently isolated organisms from hand infections?**

Staphylococci.

❑❑ **What joint is involved in a Bennett's fracture?**

The carpometacarpal (CMC) joint of the thumb.

❑❑ **What is the etiology of trigger fingers?**

Tenosynovitis in the region of the MCP joint.

❑❑ **What is the most common tumor of the hand?**

Ganglion cysts.

❑❑ **What nerve is most commonly injured in patients with an anterior glenohumeral dislocation?**

The axillary nerve.

❑❑ **T/F: Gonococcal arthritis occurs most commonly in women.**

True.

❑❑ **What is the most important characteristic of primary bone?**

It must be formed on existing surfaces.

❑❑ **What is the principle form of truncal bone growth?**

Enchondral ossification.

❑❑ **The pubic symphysis is an example of what type of joint?**

A fibrocartilaginous joint.

❏❏ **What is the most effective method for diagnosis and treatment of ligamentous knee injuries?**

Arthroscopy.

❏❏ **What are the classic P's of compartment syndrome?**

Pain, pallor, paralysis and pulselessness.

❏❏ **What is the appropriate antibiotic prophylaxis for a farming-related open tibial fracture?**

Triple-antibiotic therapy and tetanus prophylaxis.

❏❏ **What are the characteristics of a Montaggia's fracture?**

Fracture of the proximal ulna with subluxation of the radial head.

❏❏ **What is a Bankhart lesion?**

An anteroinferior glenoid labral tear.

❏❏ **What is the typical presentation of patients with osteoarthritis?**

Joint pain brought on by motion and weight bearing that is relieved with rest.

❏❏ **What are the most sensitive tests to evaluate the integrity of the anterior cruciate ligament?**

The Lachman test and the anterior drawer test.

❏❏ **What is the maximum intraoperative tourniquet time in hand surgery?**

2 hours.

❏❏ **What is the recurrence rate of osteoclastomas following curettage?**

50%.

❏❏ **What is Lasegue's sign?**

Pain and discomfort in the back when the fully extended leg of the supine patient with sciatica is raised.

❏❏ **What is the most common neurovascular injury associated with humeral shaft fractures?**

Traction injury to the radial nerve.

❏❏ **What are the advantages of internal stabilization of an open fracture?**

It minimizes soft tissue trauma, provides a stable environment for soft-tissue healing, provides pain relief, increases the likelihood of fracture healing and allows early mobilization

❏❏ **What is carpal tunnel syndrome?**

A compression neuropathy involving the median nerve as it courses deep to the transverse carpal ligament.

❏❏ **T/F: The hip is the most common site of skeletal tuberculosis.**

False.

❏❏ **What is the most common location of Pott's disease?**

The thoracic vertebral column.

❐❐ **What is the primary metabolic effect of vitamin D deficiency?**

Decreased renal tubular absorption of phosphate.

❐❐ **What is the most common location of a torus fracture?**

The distal radius.

❐❐ **Fracture of the neck of the fibula is associated with injury to what nerve?**

The peroneal nerve.

❐❐ **What is the innervation to the flexor digitorum superficialis muscle?**

The median nerve.

❐❐ **Lymphoma most commonly affects which bones?**

The femur, tibia, ilium and humerus.

❐❐ **What is the appropriate treatment for patients with chronic bacterial osteomyelitis?**

Debridement and long-term antibiotic therapy.

❐❐ **T/F: A CT scan should be performed for all patients presenting with an extremity soft tissue sarcoma.**

True.

❐❐ **What vertebra is most commonly affected in patients with spondylolisthesis?**

L5.

❐❐ **T/F: The medial meniscus is injured more frequently than the lateral meniscus.**

True.

❐❐ **What types of peripheral nerve injury are associated with extremity trauma?**

Neuropraxia, axonotmesis and neurotmesis.

❐❐ **The median nerve supplies sensation to what parts of the hand?**

The radial three and one-half digits.

❐❐ **What is the predominant type of collagen in bone?**

Type I.

❐❐ **T/F: Use of intramedullary rods for tibial fractures have results similar to those used for femur fractures.**

False.

❐❐ **Injury to which nerve will result in a Trendelenberg limp?**

The superior gluteal nerve.

❑❑ **What complications may occur if nerve repair is delayed beyond 2 weeks?**

Retraction of the nerve ends, resulting in the need for nerve grafting.

❑❑ **What are the characteristics of a Salter II fracture?**

Partial separation of the physeal plate with extension into the metaphysis.

❑❑ **Fracture of the lateral epicondyle of the humerus in children is an example of what Salter classification?**

Type IV.

❑❑ **What is the most common site of metastasis from sarcomas?**

The lung.

❑❑ **When do the clinical manifestations of torticollis first appear?**

Usually within the first 2 weeks of life.

❑❑ **What is the significance of a traumatic knee dislocation?**

It is often associated with injury to the vessels and nerves that cross the knee.

❑❑ **What are the classic signs of suppurative tenosynovitis?**

Edema and tenderness along the tendon sheath, pain with passive motion and a semi-flexed posture of the involved digit.

❑❑ **What systemic conditions are associated with carpal tunnel syndrome?**

Hypothyroidism, diabetes mellitus, obesity, acromegaly and pregnancy.

❑❑ **What is the most common site of origin for sarcomas?**

The lower extremity.

❑❑ **What is a Schmorl's node?**

Vertical disc herniation into the body of the vertebra.

❑❑ **What is the medical management of patients with rheumatoid arthritis (RA)?**

Steroids, NSAIDs and methotrexate.

❑❑ **What is the most common direction of vertebral disc herniation?**

Posterolateral.

❑❑ **Anterolateral disc herniation is usually associated with what condition?**

Spondylosis.

❑❑ **Injury to the ulnar nerve near the elbow has what effect on hand function?**

Weak adduction and abduction of digits 2 through 5.

❏❏ **What is the local recurrence rate of sarcoma following limb-sparing resections?**

10%.

❏❏ **T/F: The more unstable a fracture, the greater the cross-sectional area of the callus.**

True.

❏❏ **What test differentiates joint fluid caused by inflammatory abnormalities from that due to degenerative changes?**

The mucin clot test.

❏❏ **A herniated disc at the L4-L5 level most commonly compresses which nerve root?**

L5.

❏❏ **What is the action of the lumbrical muscles of the hand?**

Flexion of the metacarpal phalangeal (MP) joints and extension of the proximal and distal interphalangeal (PIP and DIP) joints.

❏❏ **What are the boundaries of the carpal tunnel?**

The carpal bones and the transverse carpal ligament.

❏❏ **What malignant tumor is most commonly found in the sacroccygeal area?**

Chordomas.

❏❏ **What is the expected finding on the straight-leg raising test in a patient with nerve root compression?**

Ipsilateral pain.

❏❏ **What physical findings are associated with a posterior dislocation of the shoulder?**

Loss of normal shoulder contour, posterior prominence of the humeral head and loss of external rotation.

❏❏ **T/F: Lacerations of flexor tendons have better results than lacerations of the extensor tendons.**

False.

❏❏ **What is the most common primary bone malignancy?**

Osteosarcoma.

❏❏ **What radiographic signs are associated with sarcomas?**

Extensive, poorly defined destructive lesions, often with an extraosseous component.

❏❏ **T/F: Avascular necrosis of the ulnar styloid is a common complication of Colle's fractures.**

False.

❏❏ **What is the most common cause of intertrochanteric fractures?**

A direct fall on the hip, usually in the elderly.

❏❏ **What are the most common causes of coccydinia?**

Trauma, arthritis and disc protrusion.

❏❏ **What are the characteristics of Kohler's syndrome?**

Midfoot pain with point tenderness over the navicular bone and increased density and narrowing of the tarsal navicular.

❏❏ **How long does bone remodeling usually take in an adult?**

120 days.

❏❏ **T/F: Tibial pseudoarthrosis is associated with fetal position within the uterus.**

False.

❏❏ **What are the most important prognostic factors in idiopathic scoliosis?**

The age of onset and the site of the curve.

❏❏ **What are the characteristic bone changes associated with osteitis deformans?**

Thickening, softening and deformity, followed by ossification.

❏❏ **What is the treatment of choice for patients with Paget's disease of the bone?**

Calcitonin.

❏❏ **What is the most common indication for surgical treatment of cerebral palsy?**

Spasticity.

❏❏ **What is the typical radiographic finding of osteogenic sarcomas?**

Spicules of bone within the tumor producing a sunburst appearance.

❏❏ **What is the function of the dorsal interosseous muscles?**

They spread the fingers and flex the proximal phalanges.

❏❏ **What is the earliest sign of Volkmann's ischemic contracture?**

Pain on passive extension of the fingers.

❏❏ **What is the most sensitive test for diagnosing bone metastases?**

A technetium bone scan.

❏❏ **What radiographic findings are associated with Charcot's joint?**

Marked bone destruction and loose bone fragments within abnormal joint spaces.

❏❏ **What is the long-term management of gout?**

Allopurinol.

❏❏ **What percentage of patients with long bone fractures will develop fat embolism?**

15 to 20%.

❏❏ **What is the most serious cause of limb pain after casting?**

Ischemia.

❏❏ **What are the most prominent clinical signs of fat embolism?**

Tachycardia, tachypnea, temperature elevation and mental status changes.

❏❏ **What bacterium is the most common cause of osteomyelitis in patients with sickle-cell disease?**

Staphylococcus aureus.

❏❏ **What is the typical age of presentation for a patient with Osgood-Schlatter disease?**

In the teenage years.

❏❏ **What percentage of patients with fractures of the neck of the talus will develop avascular necrosis?**

At least 50%.

❏❏ **Which gender is most commonly affected by Dupuytren's contractures?**

Males.

❏❏ **What are the histological characteristics of aneurysmal bone cysts?**

Cavernous spaces within fibrous tissue that lack an endothelial lining.

❏❏ **What organism is frequently responsible for foot infections after penetrating injuries through the sole of a sneaker?**

Pseudomonas.

❏❏ **What is the most important factor related to development of avascular necrosis of the femoral head following posterior hip dislocations?**

Delay in reduction.

❏❏ **What is the most common elbow fracture in children?**

A supracondylar fracture.

❏❏ **What serious complication may result from supracondylar fractures?**

Volkmann's ischemic contracture.

❏❏ **What is a Colle's fracture?**

Fracture of the distal radius with dorsal displacement of the distal fragment.

❏❏ **What is the most common cause of pyogenic osteomyelitis of the vertebral column?**

Hematogenous spread of Staphylococcus aureus.

❐❐ **What is the etiology of Madelung's deformity?**

Defective growth of the inner third of the distal radius.

❐❐ **What is the most common site of proximal humeral fractures?**

The surgical neck.

❐❐ **What orthopedic procedure is associated with the greatest improvement in quality of life?**

Total hip arthroplasty.

❐❐ **What is the most common etiology of malignant bony lesions in the elderly?**

Metastatic disease.

❐❐ **What type of scoliosis most often results in paraplegia?**

Untreated congenital scoliosis.

BREAST PEARLS

Nothing in life is to be feared; it is only to be understood.
Marie Curie

❑❑ **What is Mondor's disease?**

Superficial thrombophlebitis of the breast.

❑❑ **What is the most common cause of bloody nipple discharge?**

Intraductal papilloma.

❑❑ **What is the embryologic origin of the breast?**

The two ventral bands of thickened ectoderm (mammary ridges).

❑❑ **What is the appropriate initial diagnostic procedure upon identification of a palpable breast mass?**

Fine needle aspiration (FNA).

❑❑ **What is the most common cause of nonpuerperal mastitis?**

Trauma.

❑❑ **When do bacterial breast infections most commonly occur?**

During lactation.

❑❑ **What condition most commonly causes a greenish nipple discharge?**

Duct ectasia.

❑❑ **T/F: Unilateral absence of the breast (amastia) is more common than bilateral amastia.**

True.

❑❑ **What percentage of breast carcinomas occur in men?**

1%.

❑❑ **What is the most common cause of hyperprolactinemic galactorrhea?**

Primary micro- or macroadenoma.

❑❑ **T/F: Chemotherapy decreases the risk of recurrence and death from breast cancer regardless of nodal or menopausal status.**

True.

❑❑ **Breast hypoplasia is generally associated with what condition?**

Turner's syndrome (XO).

❑❑ **What are the current American Cancer Society recommendations for screening mammography?**

Women should have a base-line mammogram at 35 years of age and annual mammograms after the age of 50. Women between the ages of 40 and 50 years should consult with their physician regarding the need for regular screening.

❑❑ **What is a trunk breast?**

Marked enlargement of the areola with herniation of breast tissue into the retroareolar space. The normal contour of the breast is lost.

❑❑ **What types of glands are contained within the areola?**

Sebaceous, sweat and accessory areolar glands.

❑❑ **A 9 year old female presents with a unilateral breast lump and tenderness. What is the appropriate management?**

Reassurance.

❑❑ **What is the most common nonpathologic cause of galactorrhea?**

Mechanical stimulation, usually associated with exercise, tight clothing and sexual manipulation.

❑❑ **What is the preferred radiographic technique for confirmation of breast abscesses?**

Ultrasonography.

❑❑ **T/F: African American women have a higher incidence of fibroadenomas than Caucasian women.**

True.

❑❑ **What is the initial radiographic study for a 25 year old female with a palpable mass?**

Ultrasonography.

❑❑ **What is the average does of radiation from a routine mammogram?**

0.1 rad/exposure.

❑❑ **Which lymph nodes should be routinely examined in breast examination?**

The supraclavicular, cervical and axillary nodes.

❑❑ **Ductal proliferation is dependent on what hormone?**

Estrogen.

❑❑ **What is the leading cause of cancer-related death in women?**

Lung cancer. (Breast cancer is the second leading cause.)

❑❑ **T/F: Cystosarcoma phylloides has a high incidence of multicentricity.**

False.

❏❏ **Lobuloalveolar development depends on what hormone?**

Progesterone.

❏❏ **T/F: Obesity is a risk factor for breast cancer.**

True.

❏❏ **What is the average number of lobes in the mature breast?**

15 to 20.

❏❏ **A patient with bronchogenic carcinoma may present with what symptom relative to the breast?**

Galactorrhea.

❏❏ **What is the significance of a positive bone scan in patients with breast cancer?**

It indicates advanced disease.

❏❏ **What is the most common organism found in breast abscesses?**

Staphylococcus aureus.

❏❏ **What is the most common location of an abscess in a lactating breast?**

The upper outer quadrant.

❏❏ **What is the most common cause of breast abscesses?**

Delayed or inadequate treatment of mastitis.

❏❏ **What is the current recommended therapy for Stage I and II breast cancer?**

Modified radical mastectomy (MRM) or wide local excision with axillary dissection and radiation therapy.

❏❏ **What structure supports the breast tissue?**

Cooper's ligaments.

❏❏ **What anatomic structure defines the presence or absence of invasive breast cancer?**

The basement membrane.

❏❏ **What is the main blood supply to the breast?**

The thoracic aorta, subclavian artery and axillary artery.

❏❏ **A 45 year old female presents with a rapidly growing lesion in her right breast with ulceration of the skin near the areola. She had a normal mammogram 1 year ago and has a positive family history of breast cancer. Physical examination reveals a firm mass that replaces most of the upper outer quadrant of the breast with ulceration, with no palpable adenopathy. What is the most likely diagnosis?**

Cystosarcoma phylloides.

❏❏ **What is the treatment of choice for the above patient?**

Wide local excision or simple mastectomy.

❏❏ **T/F: Sclerosing adenosis is associated with an increased risk of breast cancer.**

True.

❏❏ **What is the most common benign breast neoplasm?**

Fibroadenoma.

❏❏ **T/F: The prognosis for breast cancer is the same in pregnant and nonpregnant women.**

True.

❏❏ **What criterion suggests malignant potential of a cyst aspirate?**

Hemorrhagic fluid.

❏❏ **What hormone receptor status is associated with the best response to hormonal therapy for women with breast cancer?**

Estrogen receptor (ER) positive with progesterone receptor (PR) negative.

❏❏ **Mastodynia is associated with consumption of what substances?**

Methylxanthines (e.g., coffee), theophylline and theobromines.

❏❏ **What are the therapeutic options for severe mastodynia?**

Vitamin E, danazol and tamoxifen.

PLASTIC AND RECONSTRUCTIVE SURGERY PEARLS

Do not resist growing old —— many are denied the privilege.
Anonymous

❑❑ **What are Langer's lines?**

Skin lines of minimal tension that generally run perpendicular to the long axis of the underlying muscle.

❑❑ **What is the embryologic origin of the dermis?**

The mesoderm.

❑❑ **T/F: Fractures of the temporal bone usually disrupt the facial nerve.**

False.

❑❑ **How does aging affect the skin?**

After about the fourth decade there is gradual thinning of the dermis, a decrease in elasticity and a loss of sebaceous material.

❑❑ **T/F: Women with silicon breast implants have an increased risk of developing breast carcinoma.**

False.

❑❑ **What is the mechanism of ossification of the craniofacial skeleton?**

Enchondral and membranous bone formation.

❑❑ **T/F: Wounds with 100,000 bacteria/gram of tissue will not support a skin graft.**

True.

❑❑ **What is the most common method of scar revision?**

Z-plasty.

❑❑ **What are the most common causes of skin graft failure?**

Hematoma, infection and inadequate immobilization.

❑❑ **How long can skin tolerate anoxia?**

Up to 24 hours.

❑❑ **What is the insertion of the medial canthus?**

The frontal process of the maxilla and lacrimal bones in the medial orbit.

❏❏ **What is telecanthus?**

Increased distance between the medial canthi.

❏❏ **What are the sources of macrocirculation to skin flaps?**

Segmental axial vessels, perforator vessels and cutaneous vessels.

❏❏ **What underlying disease processes may result in gynecomastia in adult males?**

Liver disease, pituitary abnormalities, testicular tumors and adrenal tumors.

❏❏ **What are the recommended margins for excision of basal cell cancers of the skin?**

5 mm.

❏❏ **What is the diagnostic test of choice for orbital fractures?**

CT scan with axial and coronal views.

❏❏ **What type of collagen is found in bone?**

Primarily type I.

❏❏ **What percentage of incompletely excised basal cell cancers will recur?**

One-third.

❏❏ **What are the differences between Apert's syndrome and Crouzon's syndrome?**

Children with Apert's syndrome have syndactyly of the hands, a significant incidence of cleft palate and more serious facial deformities.

❏❏ **How does delay of skin flap placement increase the success of the flap?**

It conditions the tissue to ischemia and improves vascularity.

❏❏ **What is the treatment of choice for unstable mandibular fractures?**

Open reduction and internal fixation (ORIF).

❏❏ **What histological changes occur in the skin over a tissue expander?**

The dermis thins and the subcutaneous fat diminishes while the epidermis remains unchanged.

❏❏ **What is the blood supply for the latissimus dorsi myocutaneous flap?**

The thoracodorsal vessels.

❏❏ **T/F: Initially, skin grafts survive by passive imbibition of serum.**

True.

❏❏ **Which ultraviolet waveband is responsible for sunburns as well as much of the chronic sun damage and malignant degeneration that occurs in human skin?**

UVB 315 to 290 nm.

❏❏ T/F: Split-thickness skin grafts (STSG) contract more than full-thickness skin grafts (FTSG).

True.

❏❏ What is the single most reliable test of graft viability?

Examination by an experienced physician.

❏❏ Other that sun exposure, what are the risk factors for skin cancer?

Radiation, arsenic, psoralens, atmospheric pollutants, long-standing open wounds and renal transplantation.

❏❏ What is the most common site for basal cell cancers?

The head and neck.

❏❏ What is the secondary palate?

The hard palate and the soft palate posterior to the incisor foramen.

❏❏ What are the predictors of tumor recurrence in squamous cell cancer of the skin?

The degree of cellular differentiation, the depth of tumor invasion and the presence or absence of perineural invasion.

❏❏ Squamous cell cancers in which areas of the body are prone to mestastasis?

The scalp, ears, nostrils and extremities.

❏❏ What is the single most important factor in the management of contaminated wounds?

Debridement of devitalized tissue.

❏❏ T/F: The thicker the skin graft, the greater the amount of immediate shrinkage.

True.

❏❏ What are the risk factors for melanoma?

Fair complexion, red hair, greater than 20 nevi on the body, previous diagnosis of melanoma in the individual or a first degree relative and immunodeficiency.

❏❏ What is the function of the perineurium?

Protection of the nerve trunk from stretch injury and maintenance of a constant infrafascicular pressure.

❏❏ What is the recommended excisional margin for a 3 cm melanoma?

2 cm.

❏❏ What is a Le Fort I maxillary fracture?

A maxillary fracture that extends from the piriform aperture laterally to the pterygomaxillary fissure.

❏❏ T/F: Hearing is usually impaired in patients with microtia.

True.

☐☐ **What lip defects may be closed primarily?**

Defects of up to one-third of the lower lip and one-fourth of the upper lip.

☐☐ **What is the most common cause of necrosis of a pedicle flap?**

Venous thrombosis.

☐☐ **What is the most important factor in the aesthetic outcome of lip reconstruction?**

Alignment of the vermillion border.

☐☐ **What is a stage III decubitus ulcer?**

Full-thickness skin loss and subcutaneous tissue exposure.

☐☐ **What is the most common cause of acquired ptosis?**

Dysfunction of the oculomotor nerve or sympathetic chain, usually due to trauma.

☐☐ **What are the most common sites for metastases from melanoma?**

Lymph nodes, skin and subcutaneous tissues.

☐☐ **What is the most common tumor of infancy?**

A hemangioma.

☐☐ **What are the boundaries of a unilateral cleft of the primary palate?**

From the incisor foramen anteriorly, between the canine and adjacent incisor, to the lip.

☐☐ **T/F: Children with cleft palates have an increased incidence of otitis media.**

True.

☐☐ **What is the most frequently involved suture in Crouzon's syndrome?**

The coronal suture.

☐☐ **What is the best method to minimize hyperpigmentation of skin grafts?**

Protection from UV light for one full year postoperatively.

☐☐ **What is a V-Y advancement flap?**

Closure of a rectangular defect by incising an adjacent triangle of tissue and advancing it into the defect.

☐☐ **What is the definition of a complete cleft lip?**

One that extends into the nostril floor.

☐☐ **What is the most common lymphatic malformation found in the head and neck?**

A cystic hygroma.

☐☐ What are the possible benefits of breast reconstruction?

1. Improved body image.
2. Preservation of feminine identity.
3. Elimination of external prostheses.
4. Lessened psychosocial impact of mastectomy.

NEUROSURGERY PEARLS

We know the human brain is a device to keep the ears from grating on one another.
Peter De Vries

❏❏ **What is the definition of a depressed skull fracture?**

When the inner table of the fractured skull is displaced greater than the depth of the adjacent inner table of the calvarium.

❏❏ **T/F: Hangman's fractures usually lead to quadriplegia in those who survive.**

False.

❏❏ **What are the primary diagnostic methods used to evaluate brain tumors?**

CT scan and angiography.

❏❏ **What is the most common intracranial hemorrhage following head trauma?**

A subarachnoid hemorrhage.

❏❏ **Laceration of which artery is the most common cause of epidural hematoma?**

The middle meningeal artery.

❏❏ **What is the most common pathophysiology of acute subdural hematoma?**

Disruption of bridging or cortical surface veins. Other causes include cortical contusion or laceration.

❏❏ **What is the definition of severe traumatic brain injury?**

A Glasgow Coma Scale score less than or equal to 8.

❏❏ **What percentage of the cardiac output is utilized by the brain?**

15 to 20%.

❏❏ **Below what value of cerebral perfusion pressure (CPP) is autoregulation of cerebral blood flow impaired?**

40 to 50 mm Hg.

❏❏ **T/F: An intracranial pressure (ICP) greater than 40 mm Hg is always fatal.**

False.

❏❏ **What is the most common cause of postoperative meningitis?**

Direct seeding from wound infections.

❏❏ **At what age do the majority of brain abscesses accur?**

The first 2 decades.

☐☐ **T/F: Cerebral abscesses may be treated without surgery.**

True.

☐☐ **What is the etiology of warm shock after spinal cord injury?**

Disruption of the descending sympathetic tracts that impairs vasoconstriction caudal to the injury.

☐☐ **What is the recommended duration of antibiotic therapy for brain abscess?**

6 to 8 weeks.

☐☐ **What is the Tolosa-Hunt syndrome?**

Idiopathic granulomatous inflammation of the superior orbital fissure and cavernous sinus. Patients usually present with painful ophthalmoplegia (CN III, IV and VI) and may have exophthalmos and/or chemosis.

☐☐ **T/F: Anticoagulation is contraindicated in patients with hemorrhagic venous infarction secondary to superior sagittal sinus thrombosis.**

False.

☐☐ **What are the CSF findings in a patient with a subdural empyema?**

Normal glucose, mild pleiocytosis, protein elevation and negative cultures. While CSF examination is rarely helpful, completely normal CSF makes the diagnosis unlikely.

☐☐ **What are the most common forms of disturbed water balance after traumatic brain injury?**

Diabetes insipidus, the syndrome of inappropriate antidiuretic hormone (SIADH) and cerebral salt-wasting.

☐☐ **What are the characteristics of neurogenic pulmonary edema?**

Rapid onset of decreased lung compliance without elevation of the pulmonary capillary wedge pressure (PCWP), diffuse pulmonary infiltrates and hypoxemia.

☐☐ **What is the suspected mechanism of disseminated intravascular coagulation (DIC) associated with severe brain injury?**

Activation of the extrinsic clotting cascade by release of thromboplastin from the injured brain.

☐☐ **T/F: Fixed and dilated pupils are only found with structural dysfunction.**

False.

☐☐ **Where along the course of the third nerve do the parasympathetic fibers to the ciliary ganglion divide?**

At the level of the superior orbital fissure.

☐☐ **What are the commonly employed surgical interventions for controlling medically refractory intracranial hypertension after trauma?**

Ventriculostomy, hematoma evacuation, excision of brain tissue and decompressive craniectomy.

❏❏ **What is the most common brain tumor?**

Metastases.

❏❏ **Brain lesions containing what substances are of high attenuation on unenhanced CT scan?**

Blood, calcium and melanin.

❏❏ **What are the most common locations for cerebral contusions?**

The frontal and temporal poles.

❏❏ **Where does fluid accumulation occur in patients with vasogenic edema?**

In the extracellular space.

❏❏ **What are the most common mechanisms of traumatic brain injury?**

Motor vehicle accidents (MVAs), falls and assaults.

❏❏ **What are the major arteries supplying the scalp?**

The occipital, posterior auricular, superficial temporal and orbital frontal arteries.

❏❏ **Dorsal rami of what cervical levels supply sensation to the posterior scalp?**

C2 through C4 via the greater and lesser occipital nerves as well as the greater auricular nerves.

❏❏ **T/F: Severe traumatic brain injury patients should be routinely hyperventilated.**

False.

❏❏ **What is the most common primary brain tumor?**

Glioblastoma multiforme (GBM).

❏❏ **What are the most common tumors that develop after radiation therapy to the brain?**

Meningioma and fibrosarcoma.

❏❏ **What is the most common symptom of GBM?**

Headache.

❏❏ **What layers of the vessel wall are deficient in saccular aneurysms?**

The internal elastic lamina and the media.

❏❏ **What artery is most commonly associated with an infundibulum?**

The posterior communicating artery.

❏❏ **Schwannomas of the cerebellopontine angle are usually tumors of which division of the eighth cranial nerve?**

The vestibular division.

❏❏ **What does the Schirmer test evaluate?**

Lacrimation.

❏❏ **Bilateral facial paralysis associated with progressive ascending motor neuropathy of the lower extremities and elevated CSF protein is characteristic of what clinical entity?**

Guillian-Barré syndrome.

❏❏ **How would you grade facial nerve function in a patient with facial asymmetry at rest, incomplete eye closure and minimal motion of the mouth with maximal effort?**

House Grade V.

❏❏ **Which nerves can be anastomosed to the facial nerve to improve tone and motor function?**

The hypoglossal, spinal accessory, phrenic and the contralateral facial nerves.

❏❏ **What is the average cerebral blood flow?**

50 ml/100 grams/minute.

❏❏ **What is the definition of axonotmesis?**

Loss of axonal continuity without interruption of the investing axonal tissue.

❏❏ **What conditions are suggested by the string of beads sign on angiography?**

Fibromuscular dysplasia and multifocal angiopathy.

❏❏ **What is the most common tumor of the third ventricle?**

A colloid cyst.

❏❏ **What is the most common primary benign orbital tumor in adults?**

Cavernous hemangioma.

❏❏ **What is the most common tumor of the sellar and parasellar regions?**

Pituitary adenoma.

❏❏ **What tumor markers are secreted by pineal tumors?**

Alpha-fetoprotein (AFP) and human chorionic gonadotropin (HCG).

❏❏ **What is the most common endocrine disorder associated with suprasellar extension of pineal tumors?**

Diabetes insipidus.

❏❏ **What are Lisch nodules?**

Pigmented, raised hamartomas of the iris found in more than 94% of adult patients with von Recklinghausen's neurofibromatosis.

❏❏ **What is the most appropriate treatment for symptomatic epidermoid and dermoid tumors?**

Complete surgical resection.

☐☐ T/F: Pituitary apoplexy may require emergency transphenoidal surgery.

True.

☐☐ Other than actin and myosin, what is necessary for muscle contraction?

Calcium and ATP.

☐☐ What routine part of the physical examination tests the patellar reflexes?

Stretch of the patellar ligament.

☐☐ How does a nerve cell action potential relate to the sodium/potassium channels?

Cell depolarization occurs with opening of the sodium channels, which allows an influx of sodium ions. Repolarization occurs with opening of the potassium channels.

☐☐ From what portion of the skull do chordomas most frequently arise?

The clivus.

☐☐ Extreme lateral lumbar disc herniation at L4-5 typically compresses which nerve root?

L4.

☐☐ What is the incidence of hydrocephalus following subarachnoid hemorrhage?

15 to 20%.

☐☐ Which artery and venous sinus are most often involved in a dural arteriovenous malformation?

The occipital artery and the transverse sinus.

☐☐ T/F: A normal EMG and nerve conduction study rules out carpal tunnel syndrome.

False.

☐☐ What is the most common cause of subdural empyemas in the pediatric population?

Meningitis.

☐☐ What percentage of patients with a ruptured intracranial aneurysm will have angiographic evidence of vasospasm?

More than 35%.

☐☐ What is the most common condition associated with a vein of Galen aneurysm in a neonate?

High-output cardiac failure.

☐☐ What is the appropriate management of an incidental venous angioma of the brain?

No treatment is necessary.

☐☐ What is a clay shoveler's fracture?

Avulsion of a spinous process (usually C7).

❏❏ **What is the difference in pathogenesis and treatment of acute and chronic subdural hematomas?**

An acute subdural hematoma occurs within 3 days of the incident, it is the accumulation of blood in the subdural space that causes mass effect and requires a full craniotomy. A chronic subdural hematoma is usually older than 3 weeks and can often be adequately treated with a burr hole.

❏❏ **What nerve root exits at the C4-C5 level?**

The C5 root.

❏❏ **What is the most common type of odontoid fracture?**

Type II (through the base of the dens).

❏❏ **What spinal abnormality is commonly seen in patients with rheumatoid arthritis?**

Atlanto-axial subluxation.

❏❏ **What signs and symptoms characterize benign intracranial hypertension?**

Pseudotumor cerebri, headache, blurred vision, pulsatile tinnitus, vertigo, hearing loss and papilledema.

❏❏ **What disorders are associated with endolymphatic hydrops and have symptoms that resemble Meniere's disease?**

Cogan's syndrome and otosyphilis.

❏❏ **What condition is associated with Greisinger's sign?**

Lateral sinus thrombophlebitis secondary to otitis media.

❏❏ **Reissner's membrane separates what two scala?**

The scala tympani from the scala media.

❏❏ **What is the most common inner ear malformation?**

The Mondini malformation.

❏❏ **Where is endolymph produced?**

In the stria vascularis.

❏❏ **What are the embryologic origins of the stapes?**

The superstructure is derived from the second branchial arch and the footplate originates from the otic mesenchyme.

❏❏ **Bill's bar separates what anatomic structures?**

The facial nerve from the superior vestibular nerve.

❏❏ **What organism is associated with necrotizing otitis externa?**

Pseudomonas aeruginosa.

❏❏ **What ENG findings are diagnostic of benign paroxysmal positional vertigo?**

Rotary nystagmus with latency, fatigue and subjective vertigo when the affected ear is in the lowest position during the Hallpike maneuver.

❑❑ **What is the typical physical finding in congenital cholesteatoma?**

A white middle ear mass beneath an intact tympanic membrane.

❑❑ **What is status epilepticus?**

A medical emergency defined as continuous or recurrent seizure activity without return to baseline within 15 to 30 minutes.

❑❑ **What is the definition of a subacute subdural hematoma?**

One that is more than 48 hours but less than 2 weeks old.

❑❑ **T/F: Most acoustic neuromas are inherited on chromosome 22.**

False.

❑❑ **A trauma patient with head injury does not follow commands, opens eyes only to pinching, attempts to hit you with his right arm, decerebrates on the left side and is moaning. What is his Glasgow Coma Scale score?**

Nine.

❑❑ **What are the layers of the scalp?**

Skin, connective tissue, aponeurosis, loose connective tissue and periosteum.

❑❑ **What radiologic findings are characteristic of Histiocytosis X?**

Single or multiple sharply circumscribed osteolytic lesions, most frequently found on the skull.

❑❑ **T/F: Arteriovenous malformations are the most common congenital vascular abnormalities of the CNS.**

False.

❑❑ **What is the most common tumor of the middle ear?**

A glomus tumor.

❑❑ **What is the most common site of origin of glomus tympanicum tumors?**

Jacobson's nerve.

❑❑ **In the auditory-evoked brainstem response, what is the origin of wave III?**

The cochlear nucleus.

❑❑ **T/F: The afferent fibers of the auditory nerve innervate the inner hair cells.**

True.

❑❑ **What radiographic findings occur in a Type I Arnold-Chiari malformation?**

Downward herniation of the cerebellar tonsils through the foramen magnum.

❑❑ **A patient with known HIV infection presents with seizures and two ring-enhancing brain lesions. What is the most likely diagnosis?**

Toxoplasmosis or a CNS lymphoma.

❑❑ **How often do anastamotic abnormalities occur within the circle of Willis?**

In approximately 80% of the population.

❑❑ **A young female presents 2 weeks postpartum with a severe headache and lethargy. CT scan shows the empty delta sign with some enhancement of the tentorium and cortical surface. What is the most likely diagnosis?**

Sagittal sinus thrombosis.

❑❑ **What are the major sources of brain abscesses?**

Direct extension from middle ear, mastoid and sinus infections, hematogenous spread and trauma.

❑❑ **What criteria must be met to establish the diagnosis of the Syndrome of Inappropriate Anti-Diuretic Hormone (SIADH)?**

A low serum sodium and euvolemia.

❑❑ **The corneal reflex requires which cranial nerves to be intact?**

The afferent branch of VI, V and the efferent branch of VII.

❑❑ **Through what foramen does cranial nerve VI traverse?**

The superior orbital fissure.

❑❑ **What is the treatment of choice for SIADH?**

DDAVP.

❑❑ **A child is brought to you with a dimple in his gluteal crease. You also notice a hairy patch on the child's lower back. What is the indication for an MRI of the spine?**

To determine the existence of a congenital dermal sinus.

❑❑ **In dissection of the root of the neck, what structure do you expect to find anterior to the scalene muscle?**

The phrenic nerve.

❑❑ **A trauma patient presents with an altered level of consciousness, bilateral periorbital and perimastoid ecchymosis and hemotympanum. What injury do these signs suggest?**

A basilar skull fracture.

❑❑ **What are the most common locations for hypertensive hemorrhages?**

The basal ganglia, brainstem, cerebellum, cerebrum and thalamus.

❑❑ **What is a Jefferson Fracture?**

A fracture of the ring of C1 due to axial compression.

❑❑ **T/F: There is a greater risk of infection with CSF rhinorrhea than there is with otorrhea.**

True.

❑❑ **When does denervation atrophy of muscles become irreversible?**

After 12 to 15 months.

❑❑ **What structures are contained within the carotid sheath?**

The internal carotid artery, external carotid artery and the vagus nerve.

❑❑ **A patient awakes from an abdominal procedure complaining of numbness and tingling on the medial aspect of his hand. He also feels that his hand is weak and clumsy. The patient is found to have a positive Froment's sign. What is the most likely diagnosis?**

Injury to the ulnar nerve.

❑❑ **What is the mode of cell-to-cell communication at an electrical synapse?**

Gap junction bridges.

❑❑ **What is the major advantage of a chemical synapse?**

It allows amplification and integration of input.

❑❑ **What is Seddon's classification of nerve injury?**

Neuropraxia, axonotmesis and neurotmesis.

❑❑ **During repair of a gunshot wound to the arm you note blast injury to the nervous structures. You decide to repair the nerve injuries now. How many of the injured nerves should be trimmed to make a clean anastomosis?**

Anastamosis should be delayed for at least 2 weeks to allow for the full extent of the injury to become evident.

❑❑ **The trigeminal nerve supplies innervation to what muscles?**

The muscles of mastication (the temporalis, masseter and medial and lateral pterygoid muscles).

❑❑ **Deviation of the tongue to the side indicates injury to what nerve?**

The ipsilateral hypoglossal nerve.

❑❑ **What is Wallerian degeneration?**

Degeneration of the axon distal to an injury.

❑❑ **What are the components of a chemical synapse?**

Release of pre-synaptic terminal vesicles that contain neurotransmitters. These neurotransmitters cross the synaptic cleft and bind with receptor sites on the post-synaptic cell.

❑❑ **What is the basic pathophysiology of myasthenia gravis (MG)?**

A reduction of acetylcholine receptors at the neuromuscular junction caused by an autoimmune reaction.

❏❏ **What is the treatment of choice for patients with MG?**

Thymectomy.

❏❏ **Influx of which ion is necessary for release of synaptic vesicles?**

Calcium.

❏❏ **What is the most common type of astrocytoma?**

Malignant glioblastoma multiforme.

❏❏ **What tumors most commonly metastasize to the spine?**

Lymphoma, breast, prostate and kidney.

❏❏ **A patient presents with a third nerve palsy and a recent episode of excruciating headache. What is the most likely diagnosis?**

A posterior communicating artery aneurysm.

❏❏ **A patient presents with a sudden severe headache. CT scan of the brain is normal. What further test should be performed?**

Lumbar puncture.

❏❏ **An 8 year old male was struck by a car while riding his bicycle. He presents with flaccid quadriplegia and no other injuries. Full plain x-ray evaluation reveals no fractures or spinal dislocations. What is the most likely diagnosis?**

Spinal cord injury.

❏❏ **What diagnostic test should be performed in the above patient?**

MRI of the cervical spine.

❏❏ **What contrast agent is used in MRI scanning?**

A gadolinium chelating agent (Gd-DTPA).

❏❏ **What are the indications for repair of depressed skull fractures?**

Debridement of underlying brain injury, control of subsequent edema and mass effect, prevention of post-traumatic epilepsy and control of wound contamination.

❏❏ **What are the clinical spinal cord syndromes?**

Anterior spinal cord syndrome, central cord syndrome and Brown-Sequard syndrome.

❏❏ **T/F: Older patients are more prone to sustaining subdural hematomas.**

True.

❏❏ **How can a plain skull x-ray be helpful when evaluating a traumatic epidural hematoma?**

Traumatic epidural hematomas are usually associated with a skull fracture. However, skull fractures are seen on CT scan, which is the diagnostic test of choice.

❏❏ **What measures assist in decreasing intracranial pressure and increasing systemic arterial pressure?**

Elevation of the head of the bed to 30°, intermittent drainage of CSF, hyperventilation and fluid restriction.

❏❏ **What is the most common cause of an epidural hematoma?**

A torn middle meningeal artery.

❏❏ **What is the most significant indicator of poor outcome after head injury?**

Hypotension.

❏❏ **T/F: Acute subdural hematomas are usually bilateral.**

False.

❏❏ **T/F: Traumatic intracranial contusions and hemorrhages are usually multiple and scattered, occur in the temporal and subfrontal areas and have coup and countercoup contusions.**

True. More severe head trauma can also present with intraventricular hemorrhages.

❏❏ **During the evaluation of a child with fever, you elicit a history of hydrocephalus and prior shunt placement. Chest x-ray reveals a catheter in the superior vena cava. What considerations must be taken into account?**

Shunt infection, sepsis, endocarditis and renal complications.

❏❏ **What is the Monro-Kellie doctrine in relation to intracranial pressure (ICP)?**

The cranial vault is a rigid structure that contains the brain parenchyma, blood and CSF. Normal ICP is dependent on a constant proportion of these substances. An increase in one of the parameters must be balanced by a proportional decrease in one or both of the others to maintain normal pressure.

❏❏ **Patients suffering from traumatic head injury with assumed cerebral edema are often hyperventilated. What is the physiologic rational for this treatment?**

Hyperventilation decreases intracranial pressure by decreasing $PaCO_2$, causing a decrease in pH and cerebral vasoconstriction, thus decreasing the blood volume in the cranial vault.

❏❏ **What is the most likely cause of sudden painful exopthalmos with an ocular bruit?**

A carotid-cavernous fistula.

❏❏ **T/F: A patient with transient monocular blindness and a carotid bruit is best managed by carotid end-arterectomy (CEA).**

True.

❏❏ **How much does CEA decrease the risk of stroke in the asymptomatic population?**

Up to 50%.

❏❏ **What is Cerebral Perfusion Pressure and what does it signify?**

CPP = MAP - ICP, where MAP equals mean arterial pressure. CPP represents the pressure required to push blood from the arterial tree to the venous tree in the intracranial space. If CPP is inadequate, the brain tissue will be underperfused.

❑❑ **What is the most common central disc herniation?**

Extrusion of the nucleus pulposis through the posterior aspect of the annulus and posterior longitudinal ligament into the spinal canal and/or the medial aspect of the nerve root foramen.

❑❑ **You stabilize a multiple trauma victim whose injuries include mild head injury, scalp lacerations and a femur fracture. The next morning you note a new right hemiparesis and confusion. Furthermore, his oxygen saturation has dropped to the low 90's and his urine output is declining. The patient is noted to have petechiae on his chest and in his conjunctivae. What is the most likely diagnosis?**

Fat embolism.

❑❑ **What is the pathophysiology of uncal herniation?**

An expanding mass lesion that pushes the temporal lobe medially resulting in herniation of the medial temporal lobe over the edge of the tentorial incisura, compression of the pons, midbrain and reticular activating system, loss of consciousness and, finally, respiratory and cardiac disturbances.

❑❑ **What is the difference between a communicating and a non-communicating hydrocephalus?**

A communicating hydrocephalus communicates with all of the ventricles and causes obstruction in the extra-ventricular subarachnoid space. In a non-communicating hydrocephalus, the fourth ventricle is isolated from the dilated third and lateral ventricles and causes obstruction to CSF flow.

❑❑ **A young trauma patient whose only injury was whiplash presents 1 week later with a cerebral infarct. What is the most appropriate diagnostic study?**

Angiography is the gold standard. However, MRI is becoming increasingly reliable.

❑❑ **A 76 year old male is referred to you for evaluation of urinary incontinence. During the examination you note that he has trouble ambulating. Upon further questioning you find that he has had increasing gait difficulty for several months and admits to memory loss. His history is significant for a subarachnoid hemorrhage 15 years ago. You order a head CT that shows ventriculomegaly out of proportion to brain atrophy. What is the most likely diagnosis?**

Normal pressure hydrocephalus (NPH).

❑❑ **A multiple-trauma patient is transferred to your facility with a history of head injury. The patient arrives intubated and sedated because he had a seizure prior to transport and was given 20 mg of intravenous diazepam. The patient now starts to seize again. What is the appropriate treatment?**

Phenytoin.

❑❑ **What is the treatment of choice for lacunar infarcts of the brain?**

Antiplatelet agents.

❑❑ **What complications can occur when anti-seizure medications are delivered too rapidly?**

Mortal arrhythmias and hypotension.

❏❏ **What are the CT signs of diffuse, severe brain edema that are often associated with a dismal prognosis?**

Intracranial hypertension, cerebral herniation, loss of basal cisterns, compression of the ventricles and obliteration of the third ventricle.

❏❏ **Sudden severe headache, photophobia and a stiff neck are most likely associated with what condition?**

A subarachnoid hemorrhage.

❏❏ **What is the test of choice for a patient with a suspected subarachnoid hemorrhage?**

CT scan of the head. If CT is negative but suspicion is high, a spinal tap should be performed.

❏❏ **What types of cancer most frequently metastasize to the brain?**

Lung and breast cancer are more common than melanoma simply because they occur so much more commonly in the general population.

❏❏ **What is the artery of Adamkiewicz?**

The main feeding artery to the lower half of the spinal cord.

❏❏ **An open mouth odontoid view is part of the standard evaluation of a trauma patient. This view shows the odontoid process as well as the relation of the dens to the lateral masses of the atlas. What is the significance of displaced lateral masses of C1 relative to those of C2?**

It suggests that the transverse ligament is disrupted. This is considered an unstable fracture (Jefferson fracture).

❏❏ **T/F: Enhancement after contrast administration on CT scans always implies the presence of a tumor.**

False.

❏❏ **T/F: The presence of any metal in a patient contraindicates use of an MRI scan.**

False.

❏❏ **A patient who has coarse facial features and continues to increase shoe and glove size in adulthood has what type of tumor?**

A growth hormone secreting pituitary adenoma.

❏❏ **An obese woman with hypertension, diabetes and a large deposit of fat over the lower cervical and upper thoracic spine most likely has what syndrome?**

Cushing's syndrome.

❏❏ **What is the pathognomonic appearance of an arteriovenous malformation on angiogram?**

Simultaneous appearance of arteries and veins.

❏❏ **What is the treatment of choice for intracranial aneurysms?**

Direct surgical repair.

❏❏ **What is the most common location for a spontaneous hypertensive hemorrhage in the brain?**

The putamen.

❏❏ **What is the most important initial treatment for the head injured trauma patient?**

Establishing an airway.

❏❏ **What is the classic presentation of an epidural hematoma?**

Brief loss of consciousness followed by a lucid interval with progressive loss of consciousness.

❏❏ **What are the common locations for brain contusions?**

The frontal and temporal lobes.

❏❏ **What is the optimal PaCO2 in a patient with brain injury?**

25 to 30 Torr.

❏❏ **What is the mechanism of injury in a Hangman's fracture?**

Hyperextension.

❏❏ **What is the mechanism of diffuse axonal injury?**

Rotation of the brain within the skull secondary to sudden deceleration.

❏❏ **Subdural hematomas and retinal hemorrhages in infants are pathognomonic of what syndrome?**

Shaken baby syndrome.

T/F: Brain injury usually results in hypotension.

False.

❏❏ **What are the advantages of the anterior approach for treatment of a herniated cervical disc?**

It is the most direct route and does not require manipulation of the spinal cord or nerve roots.

❏❏ **What is the most common route of CSF diversion?**

Ventriculo-peritoneal shunts.

❏❏ **What nonglial neoplasm arises from the meningothelial cells of the arachnoid villi?**

Meningiomas.

GENITOURINARY PEARLS

The mind has great influence over the body, and maladies often have their origin there.
Molière

❏❏ **What percentage of bladder and ureteral injuries occur during hysterectomy?**

75%.

❏❏ **What are the 6 types of ureteral injuries?**

Crushing injury, suture ligation, partial or complete transection, angulation of the ureter, ureteral ischemia and ureteral resection.

❏❏ **What is the most reliable means of identifying the ureter?**

Direct visualization.

❏❏ **Where do most ureteral injuries occur?**

Near the ureterovesical junction, just distal to the junction of the ureter with the uterine artery.

❏❏ **How is indigo carmine used in identifying injury to the lower genital tract?**

Indigo carmine can be given intravenously in cases of suspected bladder or ureteral injury with concomitant clamping of the transurethral Foley. This is expected to result in normal distention of the bladder with no spillage into the pelvis. Absence of dye in the bladder is indicative of bilateral ureteral obstruction. Visible dilation of the ureter is suggestive of an obstruction more distally.

❏❏ **How is the tampon test performed in trying to identify vesicovaginal and ureterovaginal fistulas?**

A tampon or sponge is placed into the vagina and methylene blue is instilled into the bladder via a transurethral Foley. If the top portion of the tampon is stained, this is suggestive of a vesicovaginal fistula. If the tampon is wet but unstained, this is suggestive of a ureterovaginal fistula.

❏❏ **What constitutes conservative management of vesicovaginal fistulas?**

Prolonged catheter drainage of the bladder, antibiotic prophylaxis and hormone replacement.

❏❏ **Where do most bladder injuries associated with vaginal hysterectomy occur?**

Near the supratrigonal portion of the bladder base.

❏❏ **What percentage of vesicovaginal fistulas are associated with abdominal hysterectomies?**

61%.

❏❏ **What is the incidence of ureteral injury with vaginal hysterectomies?**

0.12 to 4.76%.

❏❏ **Where is the ureter found in the broad ligament?**

Along the posterior sheet of peritoneum.

❏❏ **What defines the avascular perirectal space?**

The common, external and internal iliac vessels medially, the ureter laterally and the levator ani inferiorly.

❏❏ **How do the left and right ureters differ in their pelvic course?**

The left ureter enters the pelvis and crosses the common iliac artery more medially than the right.

❏❏ **How can one assess the bladder if concerned about accidentally having placed a suture through the wall?**

Cystoscopy.

❏❏ **Will ovarian tumors displace the ureter medially or laterally?**

Either type of displacement can occur, making it necessary to identify the ureter prior to beginning tumor removal.

❏❏ **What spinal segment supplies the testes?**

T10 to L1.

❏❏ **What is dialysis disequilibrium?**

Weakness, nausea, vomiting, convulsions and coma due to rapid changes in fluid and electrolyte levels.

❏❏ **What happens if distilled water is used for irrigation in genitourinary procedures?**

Visibility is the best but hyponatremia, hemolysis and convulsions leading to coma and death can occur with absorption of large amounts of water.

❏❏ **What happens when the serum sodium falls below 100 mEq/l?**

Loss of consciousness, seizures, arrhythmias, hypotension, pulmonary edema and cardiovascular collapse.

❏❏ **What is the mechanism of action of loop diuretics?**

They reduce the amount of sodium chloride reabsorbed in the ascending loop of Henle. When given as a bolus they may cause renal vasodilation.

❏❏ **What are the potential side effects of thiazide diuretics?**

Hypokalemia, metabolic alkalosis, hypercalcemia, hyperuricemia and hyperglycemia.

❏❏ **What are the short-term complications associated with transurethral resection of the prostate (TURP)?**

Absorption of hypotonic irrigation fluid leading to hyponatremia (TURP syndrome), blood loss, urinary retention and infection.

❏❏ **What symptoms are associated with bladder perforation?**

Shoulder pain, hiccuping, breathlessness, nausea, vomiting and diaphoresis.

❑❑ **What is the cardiovascular effect of immersion during extracorporeal shockwave lithotripsy (ESWL)?**

Increased cardiac output due to compression of peripheral vessels diverting blood to the central compartment.

❑❑ **What are the potential side effects of azathioprine (an immunosuppressive agent often used in renal transplant patients)?**

Bone marrow suppression, hepatotoxicity and a moderately increased requirement for non-depolarizing muscle relaxants.

❑❑ **At what level does the aorta give off the renal arteries?**

L2.

❑❑ **Behind what structure does the right renal artery course?**

The inferior vena cava.

❑❑ **What type of cell makes up the lining of the bladder?**

Transitional cell epithelium.

❑❑ **What is the most common cause of recent onset urine retention in males?**

Prostate cancer.

❑❑ **What is the most common cause of urinary retention in young males?**

Prostatic inflammation (secondary to acute urethritis and prostatitis).

❑❑ **What is the most common cause of acute right varicocele?**

Vena caval obstruction (tumor thrombus).

❑❑ **When a patient presents to the emergency room with sudden onset of severe testicular pain, what is the most likely diagnosis and why is it important to make the diagnosis quickly?**

Testicular torsion. If the torsion is not corrected within four hours, there may be irreversible damage to the testis.

❑❑ **Why are urinary tract infections more common in women?**

They have a shorter urethra.

❑❑ **What is the most common organism causing UTI?**

E. coli.

❑❑ **What organisms are most commonly associated with nonspecific urethritits?**

Chlamydia trachomatis and Ureaplasma urealyticum.

❑❑ **What is the most common site of adenocarcinoma of the prostate?**

The peripheral zone.

❏❏ **What are the best tests for detecting prostate cancer?**

Digital rectal exam and measurement of serum prostatic specific antigen (PSA).

❏❏ **What is the most appropriate therapy for men with mildly symptomatic benign prostatic hypertrophy (BPH)?**

Watchful waiting.

❏❏ **What is the most common cancer affecting the kidney?**

Renal cell carcinoma (85%).

❏❏ **What is the most common cancer affecting the kidney in childhood?**

Wilm's tumor (adenomyosarcoma).

❏❏ **Hypertension most frequently accompanies which type of renal tumor?**

Wilm's tumor.

❏❏ **A 49 year old white male with a history of tuberous sclerosis, seizures and mental retardation presents to the emergency room with systemic sepsis. A CT of the abdomen and pelvis reveals a solitary mass in the right kidney. What is the most likely diagnosis?**

Angiomyolipoma.

❏❏ **In what region of the kidney do hemangiomas most often occur?**

In the renal pelvis.

❏❏ **What is the most common tumor affecting the renal pelvocalyceal system?**

Transitional cell carcinoma.

❏❏ **What are the most common presenting symptoms of transitional cell carcinoma?**

Gross hematuria and renal colic.

❏❏ **A patient presents with a resistant urinary tract infection. He denies pain and there is no hematuria. IVP reveals markedly reduced function of the left kidney. What is the most likely diagnosis?**

Epidermoid carcinoma.

❏❏ **What percentage of prostatic nodules palpated by digital rectal exam are positive for cancer on biopsy?**

50%.

❏❏ **In a patient with prostate cancer, what test would rule out bony metastases?**

An abnormal alkaline phosphatase level.

❏❏ **What is the incidence of incontinence following prostatectomy?**

3%.

❑❑ **What is the difference in survival of prostate cancer in a patient treated by radical prostatectomy versus a patient treated with radiotherapy?**

None. The overall 5- and 10-year survivals are 75 and 60%, respectively.

❑❑ **What is the most common testicular tumor?**

Seminoma (40%).

❑❑ **Which testicular tumors are more common in men in their 20's?**

Embryonal carcinoma and teratocarcinoma.

❑❑ **Which testicular tumor produces testosterone and results in precocious puberty in children but is usually asymptomatic in adults?**

Leydig cell tumor.

❑❑ **What is the recommended postoperative adjuvant therapy for Stage A seminomas?**

27 to 36 cGy to the abdomen.

❑❑ **Which testicular tumor has the worst prognosis?**

Choriocarcinoma (it is almost always fatal).

❑❑ **Which testicular tumor is the most radiosensitive?**

Seminoma.

❑❑ **What is the most common cause of priapism?**

Injection of erection-producing agents by the patient.

❑❑ **What is the sperm count in a normal healthy male?**

Between 30 and 100 million sperm/ml with at least 70% showing purposeful motility.

❑❑ **What is the most likely diagnosis if the ejaculate lacks fructose?**

A ductal obstruction.

❑❑ **What is considered a Grade 2 renal injury?**

When there is a parenchymal laceration less than 1 cm deep without an expanding hematoma.

❑❑ **What are the possible late complications following renal injury?**

Hypertension, hydronephrosis, chronic pyelonephritis, calculus and arteriovenous fistula.

❑❑ **What is the usual treatment for injury to the lower one-third of the ureter?**

Replantation of the ureter into the bladder (neoureterocystostomy).

❑❑ **What percentage of bladder injuries are extraperitoneal?**

75%.

❏❏ **What is the most common cause of bladder injuries?**

Pelvic fracture with penetration of the bladder by bone spicules.

❏❏ **What is the treatment of choice for an intraperitoneal bladder injury?**

A two-layer closure with suprapubic drainage for several weeks.

❏❏ **Blood at the urethral meatus following blunt trauma is an indication for what diagnostic procedure?**

Urethrogram.

❏❏ **What is the initial procedure for patients with documented urethral injury?**

Cystostomy.

❏❏ **What is the most common type of urethral valve congenital anomaly?**

Type I - valves running from the verumontanum to the distal urethra (95%).

❏❏ **What are the possible complications of an unrepaired urethral valve anomaly?**

Uremia and hypertension.

❏❏ **What is the treatment for urethral valve anomalies?**

Destruction of the valves.

❏❏ **What is the most common cause of a neurogenic bladder?**

Autonomic dysfunction secondary to meningomyelocele.

❏❏ **In which sex is an ectopic ureteral orifice most common?**

Females 4:1.

❏❏ **What characteristic IVP finding indicates the presence of a ureterocele?**

A cobra-head deformity.

❏❏ **What conditions are associated with vesicoureteral reflux (VUR)?**

Posterior urethral valves, prune-belly syndrome, complete duplication of the collecting system, Ask-Upmark kidney (segmental renal hypoplasia), neurogenic bladder, bladder neck obstruction, tuberculosis, bladder infections, suprapubic and indwelling urethral catheters and bladder-urethral dysynergia.

❏❏ **What is the name for urinary reflux into the ducts of Bellini?**

Reflux nephropathy.

❏❏ **What is the most severe type of VUR?**

The golf-hole type.

❏❏ **What is the inheritance pattern of adult polycystic kidney disease?**

Mendelian autosomal dominant.

❏❏ **What are the 4-H's of adult polycystic kidney disease?**

Headache, hypertension, hematuria and heredity.

❏❏ **What percentage of premature males have an undescended testicle? Full-term males?**

30 and 4%, respectively.

❏❏ **At what age is testicular torsion most common?**

Prior to puberty.

❏❏ **What is the most common testicular tumor seen in childhood?**

Embryonal carcinoma or its yolk-sac variant.

❏❏ **What is the usual cause of a varicocele?**

Incompetent valves or obstruction of the gonadal vein.

❏❏ **What two-layered sac envelops the testis?**

The tunica vaginalis.

❏❏ **What is the most common form of the adrenogenital syndrome (CAH)?**

The 46, XX/21-hydroxylase variant (90%).

❏❏ **What is the most common fusion defect of the urethra?**

Hypospadias (1:300 male births).

❏❏ **Failure of dorsal fusion in the male urethra results in what anomaly?**

Epispadius.

❏❏ **What is the location of the renal vein in relation to the renal artery?**

The vein is anterior.

PEDIATRIC SURGERY PEARLS

Adults are obsolete children —— and the hell with them.
Theodore Geisel (Dr. Seuss)

❏❏ **What are the most common neonatal abdominal emergencies?**

Omphalocele, gastroschisis, intestinal atresias, imperforate anus, malrotation and volvulus.

❏❏ **What is gastroschisis?**

An abdominal wall defect that allows escape of the intestines from the abdominal cavity that occurs at the junction of the umbilicus and normal skin. The herniated abdominal contents are directly exposed to amniotic fluid in utero and are not protected by a layer of peritoneum.

❏❏ **Why is the prognosis for gastroschisis worse than that for an omphalocele?**

Because of the amount of time the abdominal contents spent being bathed in irritating amniotic fluid.

❏❏ **What findings are present on physical examination of neonates with congenital diaphragmatic hernia?**

Scaphoid abdomen, bowel sounds in the chest, displaced heart sounds and poor air entry.

❏❏ **What classic triad is seen in patients with a congenital diaphragmatic hernia?**

Respiratory distress, cyanosis and apparent dextrocardia.

❏❏ **What is the mortality rate of congenital diaphragmatic hernia?**

50%.

❏❏ **What therapeutic alternative(s) is/are available when persistent fetal circulation develops in a neonate with congenital diaphragmatic hernia?**

Extracorporeal membrane oxygenation (ECMO).

❏❏ **What congenital anomalies are associated with congenital diaphragmatic hernias?**

Other midline defects, including congenital heart disease (i.e., patent ductus arteriosus).

❏❏ **What bowel segments are typically involved in intestinal atresias?**

The duodenum, jejunum, terminal ileum and anus.

❏❏ **T/F: Gastroesophageal reflux is thought to be one of the primary causes of sudden infant death syndrome.**

True.

❏❏ **What is a meconium ileus?**

A small bowel obstruction caused by inspissated meconium that was never passed.

❏❏ **Bowel obstruction secondary to meconium ileus is pathognomonic for what disease?**

Cystic fibrosis.

❏❏ **What chromosomal anomaly often presents with duodenal atresia?**

Trisomy 21 (Down's Syndrome).

❏❏ **What is the age range in which pyloric stenosis is most commonly seen?**

4 to 12 weeks.

❏❏ **What classic physical finding establishes the diagnosis of pyloric stenosis?**

The olive, a palpable hypertrophic pulorus.

❏❏ **What is the most common form of congenital tracheo-esophageal fistula?**

Proximal esophageal atresia with a distal fistula.

❏❏ **In what group of anomalies is tracheo-esophageal fistula often found?**

The VATER syndrome, consisting of vertebral anomalies, anal anomalies, tracheo-esophageal fistula or esophageal atresia, renal anomalies or radial aplasia.

❏❏ **Until what age are infants obligate nose breathers?**

6 months.

❏❏ **T/F: Bilateral choanal atresia is a surgical emergency.**

True.

❏❏ **What is the most common age range for esophageal foreign bodies?**

Late infancy through early school age.

❏❏ **What are the most common esophageal foreign bodies?**

Coins.

❏❏ **What are the typical symptoms of an airway foreign body?**

Localized wheezing, dyspnea, fever and a persistent cough.

❏❏ **What types of airway foreign bodies typically produce the greatest inflammatory response?**

Food items, peanuts in particular.

❏❏ **What is the preferred maintenance fluid for children older than 6 months?**

5% dextrose in 0.45% saline.

❏❏ **Children, particularly infants, tend to have larger volumes of distribution for many drugs on a per kilogram basis than do adults. What factors contribute to this phenomenon?**

Children tend to have higher proportions of drug-to-protein binding. Protein-bound drug acts as a drug reservoir. Also, the extracellular fluid volume is greater as a proportion of total body water in children.

❏❏ **What is a direct effect of this phenomenon?**

A longer elimination half-life for many drugs.

❏❏ **Why is succinylcholine contraindicated in children with muscular dystrophy?**

They may experience acute hyperkalemia and cardiac arrest.

❏❏ **What is the hallmark of malignant hyperthermia?**

Hypermetabolism.

❏❏ **What are the most common locations for a cystic hygroma?**

The posterior triangle of the neck, axilla, groin and mediastinum.

❏❏ **What is the treatment of choice for cystic hygromas?**

Surgical excision.

❏❏ **How is croup clinically differentiated from epiglottitis?**

Croup is most prevalent in infants, whereas epiglottitis is more prevalent in toddlers and pre-schoolers. Epiglottitis is associated with high fevers, toxic appearance and a brief course before the onset of respiratory distress. Croup, however, is usually more subacute in onset with a lower temperature and WBC count.

❏❏ **What is the initial fluid resuscitation in a pediatric patient with hypotension?**

A 10 cc/kg normal saline bolus. This should be followed by a second bolus if an inadequate response is obtained. Consideration should be given to the use of blood if no response is noted after the second bolus.

❏❏ **What percentage of children less than 5 years of age will have a perforated appendicitis at the time of initial presentation?**

More than 50%.

❏❏ **What is the normal urine output for a newborn?**

1 to 2 cc/kg/hour.

❏❏ **What percentage of splenic injuries are successfully managed nonoperatively in children?**

Even splenic lacerations as severe as grade IV are usually managed conservatively.

❏❏ **What are the serum electrolyte and acid/base findings late in the course of hypertrophic pyloric stenosis?**

A hypokalemic, hypochloremic metabolic alkalosis.

❏❏ **What are the fluid and caloric requirements of an infant at birth?**

Basic fluid requirements are 65 to 100 cc/kg/day with caloric needs of 100 to 120 kcal/kg/day.

❏❏ **What is the differential diagnosis for a midline neck mass in a child?**

Thyroglossal duct cyst, dermoid cyst or adenopathy.

❏❏ **What is the most common branchial cleft anomaly?**

A second branchial cleft sinus.

❏❏ **What is the gold standard for the diagnosis of Hirschsprung's in the newborn period?**

The absence of ganglion cells in the submucosal and myenteric plexusus on rectal biopsy.

❏❏ **What is the most common presentation of Hirschsprung's disease?**

A newborn male with failure to pass meconium or chronic constipation in older infants and children.

❏❏ **What percentage of patients with cystic fibrosis present with meconium ileus as a newborn?**

10 to 20%.

❏❏ **What distinguishes a high from a low imperforate anus?**

The relationship between the rectum and the puborectalis muscle.

❏❏ **What is the initial treatment for a patient with a high imperforate anus?**

Colostomy.

❏❏ **Intraosseus access is feasible in a child until what age?**

Up to 6 years of age.

❏❏ **T/F: Malignancy is the leading cause of death in childhood.**

False. (Trauma.)

❏❏ **What are the most common presentations for patients with a Meckel's diverticulum?**

Bleeding (25-56%), obstruction (30-35%) and pain (25%).

❏❏ **What is the most common cause of death in infants with a congenital diaphragmatic hernia?**

Respiratory failure secondary to pulmonary hypoplasia.

❏❏ **What is the most common benign liver tumor in a child?**

Hemangioma.

❏❏ **What characteristics differentiate omphalocele from gastroschisis?**

Omphaloceles occur through the umbilical ring, an epithelialized sac covers the contents, the underlying bowel is normal and associated anomalies are common. Gastroschisis typically occurs through a defect in the abdominal wall to the right of the umbilicus, the bowel is uncovered and, thus, is chronically exposed to amniotic fluid and associated anomalies are less common.

❏❏ **What is the differential diagnosis of an anterior mediastinal mass in a child?**

Thymoma, teratoma, lymphoma, ectopic thyroid tissue, cystic hygroma or lipoma.

❏❏ **What is the most common soft tissue tumor in children?**

Rhabdomyosarcoma.

❏❏ **What is the most common location of a rhabdomyosarcoma in the pediatric age group?**

The head and neck region.

❏❏ **What is the rationale for correcting cryptorchidism?**

Orchiopexy is thought to enhance fertility, reduce the risk of torsion and trauma, enhance cosmesis, allow repair of the concomitant hernia and provide access for examination to exclude tumor formation.

❏❏ **What organism is most commonly implicated in post-splenectomy sepsis?**

Pneumococcus.

❏❏ **What is the most common age group for pediatric intussusception?**

Between the ages of 3 months and 3 years.

❏❏ **What is the differential diagnosis for a posterior mediastinal mass in a child?**

Bronchogenic cyst, esophageal duplication cyst, neuroblastoma, ganglioneuroma or pulmonary sequestration.

❏❏ **What are the principles of management for suspected testicular torsion?**

Rapid evaluation and treatment. If the clinical examination is inconclusive, radionuclide scanning or ultrasound can be employed to assist in diagnosis.

❏❏ **What is the surgical treatment for testicular torsion?**

Detorsion, determination of viability and fixation of both testicles.

❏❏ **What is the most common location for presentation of an extragonadal germ cell tumor in childhood?**

The saccrococcygeal region.

❏❏ **What is the differential diagnosis in a newborn that develops abdominal distention and bilious emesis?**

Malrotation, volvulus, intestinal atresias, meconium ileus or necrotizing enterocolitis.

❏❏ **What is the most common childhood malignancy?**

Leukemia.

❏❏ **What is the most common diagnosis leading to liver transplantation in the pediatric population?**

Biliary atresia.

❏❏ **What is the most common indication for splenectomy during childhood?**

Hereditary spherocytosis.

❏❏ **What is the most common intraabdominal tumor diagnosed during childhood?**

Wilm's tumor.

❏❏ T/F: A unilaterally enlarged tonsil is more likely to represent Hodgkin's disease rather than Non-Hodgkin's lymphoma.

False.

❏❏ What is the narrowest segment of the pediatric airway?

The subglottis, at the cricoid cartilage.

❏❏ What is the blood supply to the tonsil?

The facial (ascending palatine and tonsillar arteries), dorsal lingual, ascending pharyngeal and descending palatine arteries (greater palatine and lesser palatine).

❏❏ A 4 year old male presents with a slowly enlarging, firm, localized swelling over the tail of the parotid. The overlying skin is violacious and inflamed. A PPD results in a 5 mm reaction. What is the most likely etiology?

An atypical mycobacterial infection.

❏❏ A 14 year old male presents with a 1 month history of a painless submandibular mass. Examination reveals a fluctuant mass adjacent to the mandible that transilluminates. What is the most likely diagnosis?

A ranula.

❏❏ What is the treatment for the above patient?

Marsupialization into the floor of the mouth.

❏❏ A 13 year old male has recurrent nosebleeds and persistent nasal obstruction. Endoscopic nasal examination reveals a fleshy mass filling the nasopharynx. CT scan shows an enhancing mass filling the nasopharynx and pushing the posterior wall of the maxillary sinus forward. What is the most likely diagnosis?

A juvenile angiofibroma.

❏❏ What is the most common parotid mass in children?

Hemangioma.

❏❏ What is the most common malignant neoplasm of the parotid gland in children?

A mucoepidermoid carcinoma.

❏❏ What is the most common serious complication of tonsillectomy?

Bleeding.

❏❏ What is the most common primary thyroid gland neoplasm in children?

Papillary carcinoma.

❏❏ What is the most serious complication of Ludwig's angina?

Airway obstruction.

❏❏ A 15 year old male presents with complaint of a painful, swollen ear resulting from a wrestling match. Examination reveals a blottable, distorted pinna. What is the most appropriate management?

Immediate drainage under sterile conditions followed by maintenance of pressure, either by a dressing or bolster sutures and antibiotics.

❏❏ What is the most common pediatric facial fracture?

A nasal fracture.

❏❏ What is the most common cause of acute facial paralysis in children?

Bell's Palsy. However, in some series, it appears that Lyme disease may be the most common.

❏❏ What are the most common causes of inspiratory stridor in newborns?

Laryngomalacia, vocal cord paralysis and subglottic stenosis.

❏❏ What is the most common location of an airway foreign body found at bronchoscopy?

The right mainstem bronchus

❏❏ What is the significance of an omega shaped epiglottis in an infant?

It is a common finding in neonates and, as an isolated finding, is not pathologic.

❏❏ What physical features constitute the Pierre-Robin sequence?

Glossoptosis, micrognathia and cleft palate.

❏❏ What is the most common surgical approach for a pediatric tracheotomy?

A vertical incision.

❏❏ An 18 month old female has had persistent wheezing for 3 weeks despite aggressive therapy with bronchodilators. Her parents report that she had a coughing fit several days before the wheezing began, while she played on the floor. Inspiratory and expiratory chest x-rays are normal. What is the next step in management?

Rigid bronchoscopy.

❏❏ Which paranasal sinuses are present at birth?

The ethmoid and maxillary sinuses.

❏❏ What are the components of the CHARGE sequence?

Colobomata, heart defects, choanal atresia, retarded growth, genital hypoplasia and ear anomalies.

❏❏ What is the most common location of bleeding in pediatric epistaxis?

The anterior nasal septum in Kiesselbach's area.

❏❏ What are the absolute indications for operative intervention in necrotizing enterocolitis?

Pneumoperitoneum and refractory acidosis.

❏❏ **What is the typical presentation of hypertrophic pyloric stenosis?**

Nonbilious vomiting.

❏❏ **What is the survival rate of neonates with necrotizing enterocolitis colitis?**

Greater than 90%.

❏❏ **What is the appropriate treatment for a 9 year old child with hepatocellular carcinoma?**

Surgical resection and chemotherapy.

❏❏ **What is the most common renal fusion anomaly?**

A horseshoe kidney.

❏❏ **What is the inheritance pattern of infantile polycystic kidney disease?**

Autosomal recessive.

❏❏ **What are the most common complications of ureteropelvic junction obstruction?**

Hydronephrosis and urinary tract infections.

GYNECOLOGY PEARLS

It is good to rub and polish our brain against that of others.
Michel de Montaigne

❑❑ T/F: The diagnosis of high grade endometrial stromal sarcoma is usually made preoperatively.

True.

❑❑ What histologic criteria are used to diagnose leiomyosarcomas?

Hypercellularity, nuclear atypia and mitotic index. A recent study includes coagulative tumor cell necrosis as a criteria.

❑❑ What is the most frequent presenting symptom for patients with uterine leiomyosarcomas?

Vaginal bleeding.

❑❑ T/F: Leiomyosarcomas are generally solitary lesions.

True.

❑❑ What is the most common epithelial histologic subtype of malignant mixed mesodermal tumors (MMMT)?

Endometrioid.

❑❑ What physical findings are highly suggestive of MMMT?

The triad of pelvic pain, postmenopausal bleeding and tissue protruding through the cervical os.

❑❑ In a normal menstrual cycle, when does ovulation typically occur?

Day 14.

❑❑ What is the most common cause of vaginal bleeding in childhood?

A foreign body.

❑❑ What are the major categories of dysfunctional uterine bleeding?

Estrogen breakthrough, estrogen withdrawal and progesterone breakthrough.

❑❑ What is the cause of mid-cycle spotting or light bleeding?

The decline in estrogen that occurs immediately prior to the LH surge.

❑❑ Decline in what hormone heralds the onset of menses?

Progesterone.

❏❏ **What is the life-span of a normal corpus luteum in the absence of pregnancy?**

14 days.

❏❏ **What is Halban's syndrome?**

The persistence of a corpus luteum.

❏❏ **In women of reproductive age, what is the most common cause of estrogen excess bleeding?**

Chronic anovulation associated with polycystic ovaries.

❏❏ **A 24 year old female was unsuccessfully treated with oral contraceptives to control bleeding. What are the most common diagnostic possibilities?**

Complications of pregnancy, endometrial polyps and endometrial neoplasia.

❏❏ **What is the role of curettage in the treatment of dysfunctional uterine bleeding?**

To control acute hemorrhage when hormonal therapy fails.

❏❏ **What is the only estrogen currently available in oral contraceptives?**

Ethinyl estradiol.

❏❏ **What is the effect of oral contraceptives on sex hormone binding globulin?**

It increases with all pills from 180 to 390%.

❏❏ **What is the effect of oral contraceptives on total testosterone?**

It decreases from 30 to 50%.

❏❏ **What are the estrogen mediated side effects of oral contraceptives?**

Headache, nausea, breast enlargement or tenderness, fluid retention, chloasma and telangiectasia.

❏❏ **Oral contraceptive use is associated with how much of a reduction in the risk of endometrial cancer?**

54% reduction after 4 years of use with a protective effect for 15 years or more after discontinuation.

❏❏ **What is a first-degree prolapse of the uterus?**

When the cervix descends to the level of the introitus but is not seen in the introitus.

❏❏ **What is the course of the ascending limb of the uterine artery?**

Below the fallopian tube and, eventually, it anastomoses with the ovarian artery.

❏❏ **What structures form the boundaries of the broad ligament?**

The fold of peritoneum over the fallopian tube, the infundibulopelvic vessels and the hilus of the artery.

❏❏ **What are the layers of the endometrium?**

The pars basalis, zona spongiosa and the superficial zona compacta.

❏❏ **Where do primitive germ cells originate?**

In the dorsal part of the hindgut.

❏❏ **What is the karyotype of a mature teratoma?**

46 XX.

❏❏ **What is the luteoma of pregnancy?**

A benign hyperplastic reaction of ovarian theca lutein cells which may cause virilization in the mother or female fetus, although most cases are asymptomatic.

❏❏ **What surface covers the ovary?**

Germinal epithelium.

❏❏ **What ligaments support the ovary?**

The suspensory ligament at the tubal pole and the utero-ovarian ligament at the opposite pole.

❏❏ **What is the vestige of the mesonephric duct in the female?**

The Gartner's duct, which can course along the uterus, cervix and vagina.

❏❏ **What are the components of the primordial follicle?**

The oocyte with a layer of follicular cells surrounding it.

❏❏ **What is the cumulus oophorus?**

A cluster of granulosa cells around the oocyte.

❏❏ **What is Allen-Masters syndrome?**

Uterine retroversion, broad ligament lacerations, hypermobility of the cervix in all directions and enlargement and engorgement of the uterus.

❏❏ **What is struma ovarii?**

A teratoma in which thyroid tissue has overgrown other elements.

❏❏ **What is the most appropriate management for a gross cervical lesion discovered during a routine examination?**

Biopsy.

❏❏ **What percentage of adolescents with dysfunctional uterine bleeding will have a coagulation defect?**

25%.

❏❏ **What is adenomyosis?**

The presence of endometrial glands and stroma within the myometrium

❏❏ **A 5 cm carcinoma clinically confined to the cervix is assigned what International Federation of Gynecologists and Obstetricians (FIGO) stage?**

Stage Ib1.

❏❏ **What lymph node group is most frequently involved with metastatic cervical cancer?**

The external iliac group.

❏❏ **T/F: Cystoscopy and proctoscopy are necessary in the staging of all patients with cervical cancer.**

False.

❏❏ **What is the International Society of Gynecologists classification system for endometrial hyperplasia?**

Simple, complex, simple atypical and complex atypical.

❏❏ **What procedure is often considered prior to initiating radiation therapy for locally advanced cervical cancer complicated by a rectovaginal fistula?**

A diverting colostomy.

❏❏ **What pathologic findings following radical hysterectomy indicates a high risk for recurrence?**

Lymph node metastasis, surgical margin involvement and parametrial invasion.

❏❏ **What is the incidence of paraaortic lymph node metastasis for stage IIb and III cervical carcinoma?**

19 and 30%, respectively.

❏❏ **What is the intent of the pathologist when he or she makes a diagnosis of endometrial hyperplasia?**

To communicate his or her impression of the biologic potential of the endometrial proliferation to become cancer.

❏❏ **Why is endometrial hyperplasia more common at the extremes of reproductive life?**

Anovulatory cycles are more common.

❏❏ **What are the earliest signs of cytologic atypia?**

Enlarged, round nuclei with fine and evenly dispersed chromatin.

❏❏ **What is the most common presenting complaint in a postmenopausal woman with endometrial hyperplasia?**

Vaginal bleeding.

❏❏ **What factors influence the treatment of endometrial hyperplasia?**

The patient's age, amount and duration of vaginal bleeding, associated anemia, desire for future childbearing, presence or absence of cytologic atypia and the degree of cytologic atypia.

❏❏ **What life style changes are important to discuss with woman who have endometrial hyperplasia?**

Dietary and weight loss counseling, screening for diabetes mellitus and discontinuation of exogenous, unopposed estrogen.

❐❐ **What are the common side effects of GnRH therapy for endometrial hyperplasia?**

Menopausal symptoms (i.e., hot flashes and vaginal dryness), changes in the serum lipid profile, effects on the coronary arteries and bone loss.

❐❐ **What is the recommended follow-up for a woman with a histologic diagnosis of simple or complex hyperplasia without cytologic atypia?**

Endometrial sampling is recommended in 6 months.

❐❐ **What medical conditions increase the risk of endometrial cancer secondary to excess endogenous estrogen?**

Chronic anovulation, estrogen secreting ovarian neoplasms (most commonly granulosa cell and theca cell tumors), obese postmenopausal women and those with severe liver disease.

❐❐ **What is the local and distant recurrence for typical endometrial adenocarcinoma?**

20 to 30% in the pelvis, 55 to 65% at distant sites and 5 to 10% in both sites.

❐❐ **How is endometrial cancer staged?**

Surgically.

❐❐ **What percentage of endometrial carcinomas, whose only sign of extension beyond the uterus is a positive peritoneal cytology, will develop recurrent disease?**

17 to 50%.

❐❐ **What percentage of women with a diagnosis of endometrial adenocarcinoma confined to the uterus will have elevated levels of CA 125?**

12%.

❐❐ **What percentage of gynecologic oncologists would consider prescribing estrogen replacement for a woman treated for stage 1 grade 1 endometrial cancer?**

83%.

❐❐ **What is a Walthard nest?**

A benign inclusion cyst created in the fallopian tube by invagination of the tubal serosa.

❐❐ **What is salpingitis isthmica nodosa?**

A localized diverticulosis of the isthmic portion of the fallopian tube.

❐❐ **What percentage of primary malignancies of the female genital tract arise from the fallopian tubes?**

0.2 to 0.5%.

❐❐ **What is the most common primary malignant neoplasm of the fallopian tube?**

Papillary serous adenocarcinoma.

❑❑ **What triad of symptoms is associated with fallopian tube malignancies?**

Profuse clear or serosanguinous vaginal discharge (hydrops tubae profluens), pelvic pain and a pelvic mass.

❑❑ **A tubal lesion consisting primarily of trophoblastic proliferation and hydropic villi represents what type of fallopian tube tumor?**

An ectopic molar pregnancy.

❑❑ **What is the role of cytoreductive surgery?**

For residual tumor mass less than 1 cm.

❑❑ **What are the methods of spread of tubal carcinomas?**

Transcoelomic exfoliation of cells via the fallopian tube, direct extension and lymph/vascular invasion.

❑❑ **What percentage of gynecologic malignancies originate on the vulva?**

3 to 5%.

❑❑ **What risk factors have been linked with vulvar cancer?**

Advancing postmenopausal age, hypertension, diabetes, obesity and smoking.

❑❑ **T/F: Lichen sclerosis has been proven to be a precursor of and leads to invasive vulvar cancer.**

False.

❑❑ **What is a Stage IA vulvar cancer?**

The tumor is confined to the vulva or perineum, it is 2 cm or less in greatest dimension, there are no nodal metastases and stromal invasion is less than or equal to 1 mm.

❑❑ **What are the most common histologic subtypes of vulvar neoplasms?**

Epidermoid (squamous cell), melanoma, sarcoma, basal cell and Bartholin gland.

❑❑ **What underlying malignancy must be ruled out when Paget's disease of the vulva is diagnosed?**

Adenocarcinoma of the vulva.

❑❑ **What is the most frequent primary vulvar sarcoma?**

Leiomyosarcoma.

❑❑ **What is the incidence of positive lymph node involvement in T2 lesions?**

45%.

❑❑ **What is a merkel-cell tumor?**

A neuroendocrine vulvar tumor of the skin that resembles small-cell carcinomas of neuroendocrine type in other body sites and is associated with frequent lymph node metastasis and a poor prognosis.

❑❑ **What HPV subtype has been associated with verrucous carcinomas of the vulva?**

Type 6.

❏❏ **What are the subtypes of vulvar malignant melanoma?**

Superficial spreading, nodular and acral lentiginous.

❏❏ **What is the survival rate with positive deep pelvic nodes in vulvar cancer?**

20%, regardless of stage.

❏❏ **T/F: Adjuvant chemotherapy improves survival in patients with vulvar carcinoma.**

False.

❏❏ **What is the overall rate of recurrence in treated vulvar cancer?**

25%.

❏❏ **What vaginal tumor presents as a mass of grape-like nodules, most commonly in the first 2 years of life?**

Embryonal rhabdomyosarcoma (sarcoma botryoides).

❏❏ **What have post-operative spindle cell nodules on the vulva been confused with?**

Leiomyosarcomas.

❏❏ **Which vulvar cancer has a predilection for hematogenous spread?**

Vulvar sarcomas.

❏❏ **T/F: Primary cancer of the vagina is one of the rarest of the malignant processes in the human body.**

True.

❏❏ **What is the primary mode of therapy for vaginal cancer?**

Radiation therapy.

❏❏ **What is the most frequent location of a primary vaginal carcinoma?**

The upper third and posterior wall of the vagina.

❏❏ **What is the typical radiation treatment plan for larger stage I vaginal cancers?**

Whole pelvis external radiation with 4,000 to 5,000 cGy and an interstitial implant delivery of 3,000 cGy.

❏❏ **What is the stage of a vaginal cancer that has spread to the pelvic sidewall?**

Stage III.

❏❏ **What precursor lesion is found in clear cell adenocarcinoma of the vagina?**

Adenosis.

❏❏ **What has clear cell carcinoma of the vagina and cervix been thought to be associated with?**

In utero DES exposure.

❑❑ **What is the overall survival rate for patients with vaginal melanomas?**

15%.

❑❑ **What histologic finding is associated with clear cell adenocarcinomas?**

Hobnails.

❑❑ **Where are clear cell adenocarcinomas of the genital tract most commonly located?**

In the ectocervix and upper anterior wall of the vagina.

❑❑ **What is the overall survival rate of clear cell adenocarcinoma of the vagina /cervix?**

80%.

❑❑ **T/F: Laparoscopic procedures can be done during pregnancy.**

True.

❑❑ **What is the best time to perform elective surgery during pregnancy?**

All elective surgeries should be postponed until after delivery. Urgent surgeries are preferably deferred until the second or third trimester.

❑❑ **What are the major prognostic factors in vulvar cancer?**

Tumor size, depth of tumor invasion, nodal spread and distant metastases.

❑❑ **What is the frequency of pelvic recurrence for Stage IV vaginal cancer?**

58%.

❑❑ **What muscles form the floor of the pelvis?**

The levator ani (pubococcygeus, puborectalis, iliococcygeus and coccygeus muscles).

❑❑ **What are the boundaries of the urogenital hiatus?**

The pubococcygeus muscle laterally and the symphysis pubis anteriorly.

❑❑ **What is the cul de sac of Douglas?**

The peritoneal recess posterior to the uterus.

❑❑ **What structure demarcates the obstetric or true pelvis, from the false pelvis?**

The pelvic brim.

❑❑ **What is the blood supply to the pelvis?**

The internal iliac arteries and the middle sacral artery.

❑❑ **What is the normal pH of the vagina?**

3.8 to 4.4.

❏❏ **What organisms are most commonly associated with PID?**

N. gonorrhea and chlamydia.

❏❏ **What is thought to be the cause of endometriosis?**

Retrograde menstruation.

❏❏ **Where is endometriosis most commonly found?**

On the ovary.

❏❏ **What is the most likely diagnosis of a women presenting with irregular menses and occasional extended intervals of amenorrhea?**

Dysfunctional uterine bleeding.

❏❏ **What is the most common viral infection of the vulva and vagina?**

Condyloma acuminatum.

❏❏ **What percentage of patients with pelvic inflammatory disease become infertile?**

10%.

❏❏ **What is a Nabothian cyst?**

A mucous inclusion cyst of the cervix (usually asymptomatic and harmless).

❏❏ **What is the treatment for Stage 1A or 1B ovarian cancer?**

Total abdominal hysterectomy and bilateral salpingoopherectomy (TAH/BSO).

❏❏ **What is the overall 5-year survival rate for patients with ovarian cancer?**

37%.

❏❏ **What are the risk factors for carcinoma of the cervix?**

Multiple sexual partners, early age at first intercourse and early first pregnancy.

❏❏ **By what route do cervical cancers usually spread?**

Predominantly by lymphatic channels.

❏❏ **What stage(s) of cervical cancer is/are associated with a risk of pelvic lymph node spread?**

Stage IB and IIA.

❏❏ **T/F: When performing a radical hysterectomy for cervical cancer, oopherectomy must also be performed.**

False.

❏❏ **What are the risk factors for vulvar carcinoma?**

Older age, smoking, previous squamous cell carcinoma of the cervix or vagina, chronic vulvar dystrophy, and immunocompromise.

❏❏ **Cancer of what area is associated with human papilloma virus?**

Vulvar carcinoma.

❏❏ **What is the treatment of choice for vulvar carcinoma?**

Radical vulvectomy with inguinal lymphadenectomy.

❏❏ **What are the indications for dilation and curettage?**

Removal of an endometrial polyp or hydatid mole, termination of pregnancy/incomplete abortion, removal of retained placental tissue and relief of profuse uterine hemorrhage.

❏❏ **What major complication is associated with dilation and curettage?**

Perforation

HEMATOLOGY AND ONCOLOGY PEARLS

Fever, the eternal reproach to the physician.
John Milton

❏❏ **Epstein-Barr virus is associated with what cancers?**

Nasopharyngeal cancer and Burkitt's lymphoma.

❏❏ **What are the major antibodies in tumor immunity?**

IgA and IgE.

❏❏ **In what conditions is PSA elevated?**

Benign prostatic hypertrophy (BPH) and prostatic carcinoma.

❏❏ **What are restriction enzymes?**

Nucleases that cut DNA only at specific sequences of nucleotides.

❏❏ **What is Grey Turner's sign?**

Flank ecchymosis, classically secondary to hemorrhagic pancreatitis.

❏❏ **T/F: Symptomatic metastatic breast carcinoma in an indication for palliative surgery.**

True.

❏❏ **Alpha-fetoprotein (AFP) is found in what fetal tissues?**

The gastrointestinal tract, liver and yolk sac.

❏❏ **Radiation targets what part of the cell?**

The nucleus.

❏❏ **What are the mechanisms by which proto-oncogenes may be activated?**

Mutation, amplification or translocation.

❏❏ **T/F: Patients with hairy-cell leukemia may be treated by splenectomy.**

True.

❏❏ **T/F: Cobalt-60 is considered low-energy.**

False.

❏❏ T/F: Low-energy x-rays have a skin-sparing effect.

False.

❏❏ When do the chemical changes within cells occur after radiation therapy?

Within seconds.

❏❏ Where is human chorionic gonodotropin (HCG) produced?

The placenta (the synctiotrophoblast).

❏❏ As tissue factor is released from injured cells, which coagulation factor does it complex with to activate the extrinsic pathway?

Factor VII.

❏❏ Activated factor IX, (IXa), in combination with which two cofactors, activates factor X on the surface of platelets?

Ionized calcium and factor VIIIa.

❏❏ How does activated protein C work?

It inactivates factors Va and VIIIa.

❏❏ What protein is a cofactor for protein Ca?

Protein S.

❏❏ T/F: The latency period in carcinogenesis is dose-dependent.

True.

❏❏ How does antithrombin III work?

It binds to thrombin, preventing the activation of fibrinogen, factor V, factor VII and the activation and aggregation of platelets. Antithrombin III also inhibits factors IXa, Xa and XIa.

❏❏ What is the main fibrinolytic enzyme?

Plasmin.

❏❏ In what form is factor D released during physiologic clot formation?

Dimeric form (D-dimers).

❏❏ What exogenous factor activates plasminogen?

Streptokinase.

❏❏ What type of blotting technique is used to analyze DNA structure?

A Southern blot.

❏❏ Circulating neutrophils and monocytes interact with endothelial cells through which two molecules?

P-selectin and E-selectin.

❏❏ **What systemic chemotherapeutic agent is used in the treatment of bladder cancer?**

Flutamide.

❏❏ **What are proto-oncogenes?**

Proteins that are capable of inhibiting oncogenes.

❏❏ **T/F: Changing from bovine derived heparin to porcine derived heparin is sufficient therapy for a patient with heparin-induced thrombocytopenia.**

False.

❏❏ **What are the molecular events in heparin-induced thrombocytopenia?**

It is believed to be caused by a heparin-dependent IgG platelet antibody that causes aggregation of platelets when exposed to heparin.

❏❏ **CEA is an example of what type of tumor marker?**

An oncofetoprotein.

❏❏ **What are the common causes of acquired antithrombin III deficiency?**

Liver disease, malignancy, nephrotic syndrome, DIC, malnutrition or increased protein catabolism.

❏❏ **What is the appropriate anticoagulation therapy for a patient with antithrombin III deficiency?**

Fresh frozen plasma (FFP) can be used as a source of antithrombin III when heparin is necessary, followed by anticoagulation with sodium warfarin. Additionally, antithrombin III concentrates are available.

❏❏ **How does sodium warfarin (Coumadin) work as an anticoagulant?**

It prevents the reduction of vitamin K once it has functioned as a cofactor for the (carboxylation of factors II, VII, IX and X).

❏❏ **What other factors does coumadin inhibit?**

Protein C and S.

❏❏ **T/F: Resistance to activated protein C is more common than protein C deficiency.**

True. It has been reported that 40% of patients who present with idiopathic venous thrombosis have this disorder.

❏❏ **What is involved in a Phase I drug trial?**

It determines the maximally tolerated dose (MTD) and outlines the toxicity profile.

❏❏ **What is the antiphospholipid syndrome?**

The presence of antiphospholipid antibody or the lupus anticoagulant along with any or all of the following: recurrent thromboses, recurrent fetal losses, thrombocytopenia or livido reticularis.

❏❏ **What is the treatment for Hodgkin's disease?**

Combination chemotherapy, such as nitrogen mustard, vincristine (Oncovin), procarbazine and predinsone (MOPP) or MOPP/ABV (adriamycin, bleomycin and vinblastine).

❑❑ **What is the molecular abnormality in hemophilia A?**

An inherited sex-linked recessive deficiency of factor VIII.

❑❑ **What are the clinical manifestations of hemophilia A?**

Bleeding into joints and muscles, epistaxis, hematuria and bleeding after minor trauma

❑❑ **T/F: Hemophilia A is clinically distinguishable from hemophilia B.**

False.

❑❑ **What is carcinoma-in-situ?**

A malignant neoplasm that has not yet invaded the basement membrane.

❑❑ **What is the molecular abnormality in Von Willebrand's Disease?**

Reduction of factor VIII activity and vWF-factor VIII complex, resulting in an inability of platelets to bind to collagen.

❑❑ **What is the most common complication of massive transfusion?**

Dilutional thrombocytopenia.

❑❑ **What is the dose limiting toxicity associated with Cisplatin?**

Nephrotoxicity.

T/F: Anticancer drugs can kill a fixed number of tumor cells per dose.

False.

❑❑ **What are the types of bone marrow transplantation?**

Autologous, syngeneic and allogeneic.

❑❑ **What is vincristine belly?**

Constipation caused by autonomic neuropathy secondary to vincristine.

❑❑ **What is the most common secondary malignancy associated with the use of chemotherapy?**

Acute nonlymphocytic leukemia.

❑❑ **What is the best way to avoid cisplatin induced renal toxicity?**

Aggressive pretreatment hydration.

❑❑ **What is the growth fraction of a tumor?**

The number of cells actively involved in cell division.

❑❑ **Methotrexate is specific for what phase of the cell cycle?**

The S phase.

❑❑ **What drugs are used for prevention of hypersensitivity reactions associated with paclitaxel?**

Corticosteroids and H1 and H2 blockers.

❑❑ **What is the dose limiting toxicity associated with vincristine?**

Neurotoxicity.

❑❑ **What is the mechanism of action of 5-fluorouracil (5-FU)?**

Competitive inhibition of thymidylate synthetase.

❑❑ **Cisplatin is associated with depletion of what electrolytes?**

Potassium, magnesium and calcium.

❑❑ **T/F: Fever is a frequent side effect of bleomycin.**

True.

❑❑ **What is the mechanism of action of melphalan?**

It is an alkylating agent.

❑❑ **Ototoxicity associated with cisplatin typically involves what part of the audible range?**

High frequencies.

❑❑ **T/F: Arthralgia is a side effect associated with paclitaxel.**

True.

❑❑ **What is the mechanism of action of Topotecan?**

It is a topoisomerase I inhibitor.

❑❑ **Diagnosis of the syndrome of inappropriate antidiuretic hormone (SIADH) associated with cyclophosphamide is made by what lab findings?**

Hyponatremia with less than maximally dilute urine.

❑❑ **T/F: Adriamycin is primarily excreted by the kidneys.**

False.

❑❑ **What is the mechanism of action of Etoposide?**

It is an inhibitor of topoisomerase II.

❑❑ **What is Leucovorin?**

Folinic acid. It is used to prevent toxicity from high-dose methotrexate.

❑❑ **T/F: Alopecia is a frequent side effect of vinblastine.**

True.

❏❏ **What is the mechanism of action of bleomycin?**

DNA scission with inhibition of DNA ligase.

❏❏ **How is vincristine primarily excreted?**

By the liver.

❏❏ **What is the longest phase of the active cell cycle?**

G1.

❏❏ **What is the mechanism of action of hydroxyurea?**

Inhibition of ribonucleotide reductase.

❏❏ **T/F: Dermatitis and nail loss are frequent toxicities of bleomycin.**

True.

❏❏ **What is the initial treatment for ifosfamide induced hemorrhagic cystitis?**

Hydration and diuresis.

❏❏ **What is the most common neurologic side effect associated with cisplatin?**

Peripheral neuropathy of the hands and feet.

❏❏ **What is the dose-limiting toxicity associated with DTIC (dacarbazine)?**

Myelosuppression.

❏❏ **What is the purpose of maintaining a patient's urine pH below 7.0 when administering high dose methotrexate?**

To minimize renal toxicity.

❏❏ **T/F: Antiemetic drugs for chemotherapy-induced nausea are most effective when given prior to chemotherapy.**

True.

❏❏ **Tamoxifen is used to antagonize the effect of estrogen on breast cancer, yet may induce endometrial bleeding and cancer. Why?**

Tamoxifen is a mixed estrogen agonist/antagonist, depending on the target tissue.

IMMUNOLOGY AND TRANSPLANTATION PEARLS

The wise man mourns less for what age takes away then what it leaves behind.
William Wordsworth

❐❐ **T/F: An allograft is a tissue or organ graft between two individuals of the same species.**

True.

❐❐ **What is a syngeneic graft?**

A graft between identical twins.

❐❐ **What chromosome contains the major histocompatibility complex (MHC)?**

Chromosome 6.

❐❐ **What are the human gene products of the MHC?**

The human leukocyte antigens (HLA).

❐❐ **What cells have HLA Class I molecules?**

All nucleated cells.

❐❐ **What cells have HLA Class II molecules?**

Macrophages, dendritic cells, B cells and activated T cells.

❐❐ **T/F: Interferons (IFN-alpha, IFN-beta and IFN-gamma) induce increased expression of Class I molecules.**

True.

❐❐ **What cells produce IFN-gamma?**

Lymphocytes.

❐❐ **What are the methods of determining the degree of histocompatibility between donor and recipient?**

MHC matching and mixed lymphocyte culture (MLC).

❐❐ **What is the MLC test (functional typing)?**

Lymphocytes of the recipient are mixed with those of the donor. If there are significant antigenic differences, they will respond by proliferation with transformation into blast cells, DNA synthesis and mitosis.

❑❑ **What is the result of a reaction between IgG or IgM and cell-bound antigen?**

A Type II hypersensitivity reaction.

❑❑ **What cells give rise to the cellular components of the immune system?**

The pleuropotential bone marrow stem cells.

❑❑ **What regulates production of the lineages of the stem cell?**

Cytokines.

❑❑ **What are the critical cytokines that influence lineage maturation?**

Granulocyte-macrophage colony stimulating factor (GM-CSF), interleukin-1 (IL-1) and erythropoietin.

❑❑ **What is the clinical use of erythropoietin?**

It decreases the need for transfusion in patients with anemia secondary to renal failure.

❑❑ **Where do progenitor lymphoid cells mature into T cells?**

In the thymus.

❑❑ **What organs are considered primary lymphoid organs?**

The thymus and the bone marrow.

❑❑ **What cells are responsible for humoral immunity?**

B cells.

❑❑ **T/F: Peripheral B cells are fully immunocompetent.**

True.

❑❑ **What constitutes the T-cell receptor complex (CD3)?**

The T cell's membrane bound T-cell receptor (TCR) and associated transmembrane proteins.

❑❑ **What T cell cluster of differentiation (CD) antigen lyses target cells and kills cells infected with virus?**

CD8.

❑❑ **What is required for a lymphocyte to become sensitized?**

An accessory antigen-presenting cell (APC) of the monocyte-macrophage line.

❑❑ **What other function do APCs perform?**

They secrete cytokines (i.e., IL-1) that enhance the T cell response in the immediate vicinity.

❑❑ **What are the functions of IL-1 with regard to the immune cellular response?**

It fosters the appearance of IL-2 receptors (IL2R) and stimulates IL-2 secretion from antigen-sensitive CD4 and helper T cells.

❑❑ **What do cytotoxic CD8 and T cells require to develop lymphocyte-mediated cytotoxicity?**

T-helper cytokines.

❑❑ **What morphologic differentiation accompanies B cell proliferation?**

B cells become antibody-producing plasma cells.

❑❑ **What cells do Class I alloantigens preferentially stimulate?**

CD8 and T-helper cells.

❑❑ **T/F: Circulating antibody is an obligatory participant in the rejection of solid tissue allografts.**

False.

❑❑ **How do antibodies activate the complement pathway?**

When an antibody binds to antigen, the antibody undergoes a conformational change that activates the constant (Fc) end of the antibody, which then triggers complement activation.

❑❑ **T/F: Cytokines primarily act in an endocrine manner.**

False.

❑❑ **How do cytokines exert their effect?**

They bind to cell surface receptors and cause transmembrane signal transduction. This results in increased cellular RNA, protein synthesis and, ultimately, altered cell behavior.

❑❑ **What are the macrophage-derived cytokines?**

IL-1, Il-6 and TNF-alpha.

❑❑ **What are the effects of IL-1?**

Fever, release of hepatic acute-phase proteins and release of neutrophils, ACTH, cortisol and insulin. The effects of IL-1 on endothelial cells include increased leukocyte adherence, prostaglandin release and hypotension.

❑❑ **What complement pathway is the most important for immune reactions?**

The classic pathway.

❑❑ **What are the actions of C5a?**

It is a potent chemotactic factor, stimulates histamine release from mast cells, attracts neutrophils and it liberates lysosyme from neutrophils.

❑❑ **T/F: Complement is capable of self-amplification.**

True.

❑❑ **What is the initiating factor of the extrinsic pathway of the clotting system?**

Release of tissue thromboplastin.

❏❏ **What activates Hageman factor (factor XII)?**

Antigen-antibody complexes.

❏❏ **What are the biologic activities of kinins?**

Chemotaxis of PMNs, smooth muscle contraction, dilatation of peripheral arterioles and increased capillary permeability.

❏❏ **What series of events follows allograft transplantation in an unsensitized patient?**

1. Perivascular infiltration of round cells.
2. Deposition of antibody and complement near the capillaries.
3. Release of several mediators of inflammation and cell damage.
4. Fixation of complement.
5. Increased capillary permeability, interstitial edema and infiltration of PMNs.
6. Fibrin deposition, which decreases perfusion and prevents function.

❏❏ **What repair process is elicited by endothelial cell damage?**

Accelerated atherosclerosis.

❏❏ **What are the methods by which immunosuppressive agents suppress the rejection response?**

Destruction of immunocompetent cells or inhibition of differentiation and proliferation of these cells.

❏❏ **Most immunosuppressive agents are directed at what cells?**

T-helper cells.

❏❏ **What is the mechanism of action of cyclosporin?**

It inhibits T-cell activation and maturation.

❏❏ **What is the mechanism of action of OKT3?**

It binds to the CD3 portion of the T-Cell receptor.

❏❏ **What immunosuppressive agents act on the G0 phase of the cell cycle?**

OKT3, FK 506 and CsA.

❏❏ **On what phase of the cell cycle does azathioprine act?**

The S phase.

❏❏ **How do antimetabolites suppress the immune response?**

They inhibit enzymes in metabolic pathways or they are incorporated during synthesis to produce faulty molecules.

❏❏ **What are the common antimetabolites used for chronic immunosuppression?**

Purines, pyrimidines and folic acid analogues.

❏❏ **Why are alkylating agents only used in patients receiving a bone marrow transplant?**

They are too toxic. However, they are occasionally used as a substitute for azathioprine (AZ).

❏❏ **What is the primary toxic effect of AZ?**

It is toxic to the bone marrow, resulting in leukopenia.

❏❏ **What is the role of folic acid antagonists in immunosuppression?**

They inhibit dihydrofolate reductase and prevent the conversion of folic acid to tetrahydrofolic acid. Thus, they inhibit synthesis of DNA, RNA and certain coenzymes.

❏❏ **When are alkylating agents most effective?**

When given just before and during stimulation of the immunocompetent cells.

❏❏ **What combination of drugs provides the most effective immunosuppression with the fewest side effects?**

Cyclosporine, prednisone and/or AZ.

❏❏ **What is the mechanism of action of cyclosporine?**

It is a cyclic peptide produced by a fungus that specifically suppresses T cells and inhibits production of IL-2.

❏❏ **T/F: Cyclosporine is primarily excreted in the urine.**

False. It is primarily excreted in the bile.

❏❏ **What is the advantage of cyclosporine over antimetabolites?**

It does not cause myelosuppression.

❏❏ **What are the primary toxic effects of FK 506?**

Anorexia and nephrotoxicity.

❏❏ **How does rapamycin (RAPA) affect the immune response?**

It strongly inhibits IL-4 and IL-2 driven proliferation by blocking the ability of the IL-2 receptor to induce signal transduction.

❏❏ **What is the effect of large doses of corticosteroids on lymphocytes?**

Destruction and lysis.

❏❏ **What other immune cells are affected by corticosteroids?**

Macrophages, neutrophils and monocytes.

❏❏ **What is the most important mode of cellular damage from radiation?**

Production of scattered breaks in the deoxyribose-phosphate backbone of DNA.

❏❏ **In what stage(s) of the cell cycle is radiation most effective?**

The M and G2 phase. (Lymphocytes are also sensitive in the G0 phase.)

❏❏ **Antilymphocyte globulins (ALG) mainly affect what immune cells?**

T cells.

❏❏ **What are the common side effects of monoclonal antibodies?**

Fever, chills, nausea, diarrhea and aseptic meningitis.

❏❏ **What is the most common cause of death in transplant recipients?**

Infection.

❏❏ **The majority of deaths in transplant recipients are due to what organisms?**

Candida albicans and aspergillus.

❏❏ **What are the most common viral organisms causing rejection in renal transplant patients?**

The herpes group DNA viruses.

❏❏ **What percentage of renal transplant patients are infected with cytomegalovirus (CMV)?**

50 to 90%.

❏❏ **T/F: Standard patient isolation precautions decrease the number of opportunistic infections.**

False.

❏❏ **What are the most frequent malignancies seen in transplant patients?**

Those that are common to immunosuppressed patients. Most are epithelial or lymphoid in origin (i.e., carcinoma in situ of the cervix, carcinoma of the lip, squamous or basal cell carcinoma of the skin and B cell lymphoma).

❏❏ **What is the incidence of lymphoma in transplant recipients?**

350 times the average population.

❏❏ **What percentage of transplant patients with lymphoma have brain involvement?**

50%.

❏❏ **What is thought to be the etiology of lymphoma in transplant patients?**

Infection with Ebstein-Barr virus (EBV) (lymphoproliferative disease) (LPD).

❏❏ **What type of corneal transplant is used for patients with corneal opacity and does not involve the full thickness of the cornea?**

Lamellar keratoplasty.

❏❏ **What is thought to be the reason for the long-term success of corneal transplants?**

Corneal grafts are in a privileged location in which they remain effectively isolated from the immune system.

❏❏ **What are the indications for bone implants?**

To hasten the healing of defects and cavities, to supplement bony union of delayed healing and to reconstruct major skeletal defects.

❏❏ **T/F: Cartilage grafts can be transferred between individuals of different genetic backgrounds without immunosuppressive therapy.**

True.

❏❏ **What is the critical period of ischemia after which extremity replantation is unsuccessful?**

There is no definite time, however, it appears that successful replantation of a limb can occur after 12 hours of ischemia and up to 36 hours for a finger.

❏❏ **Why are more distal amputations able to tolerate longer periods of ischemia?**

Because there is less ischemia-sensitive muscle.

❏❏ **T/F: In extremity replantation, bone fixation is carried out prior to vascular anastamosis.**

True.

❏❏ **T/F: Nerve grafts/anastamoses can be delayed and performed in a secondary operation.**

True.

❏❏ **T/F: Motor nerve recovery is more successful in the ulnar nerve than in the median nerve.**

False.

❏❏ **T/F: Muscle debridement is carried out after the blood supply is restored.**

True. The viability of muscle is better ascertained after the blood supply is re-established. However, grossly devitalized tissue must be debrided prior to replantation.

❏❏ **What is the treatment of acidosis following replantation?**

Bicarbonate and mannitol.

❏❏ **What are the most commonly used musculocutaneous grafts for wound coverage?**

The rectus abdominus and latissimus dorsi.

❏❏ **What results when mature T cells accompany a donor graft?**

The graft-versus-host (GVH) reaction.

❏❏ **What are the target tissues of donor T cells in the GVH reaction?**

The skin, liver and gastrointestinal tract.

❏❏ **What factors are essential for the existence of GVH?**

A recognizable antigen difference between the donor and host, immunocompetent T cells and a relative immunocompromise of the recipient.

❏❏ **How is the diagnosis of GVH reaction confirmed?**

Skin biopsy.

❏❏ **T/F: A missed diagnosis of GVH reaction is almost universally fatal.**

True.

☐☐ **What are the indications for autotransplantation of the parathyroid?**

Severe secondary hyperparathyroidism, primary generalized parathyroid hyperplasia and unintentional removal of parathyroid tissue.

☐☐ **What is the most frequent site of parathyroid transplantation?**

The volar forearm.

☐☐ **What is the most common indication for renal transplantation?**

Diabetic renal failure.

☐☐ **T/F: Islet cell grafts are less antigenic than whole organ grafts.**

False.

☐☐ **T/F: Islet cell graft rejection is accelerated compared to whole organ grafts.**

True. (Especially is diabetics, secondary to autoimmunity.)

☐☐ **Why is there such interest in islet cell grafts when they have such dismal success rates?**

When the rejection reaction is overcome, there is no better way to improve the vascular and neurologic lesions of diabetes.

☐☐ **What is the major technical concern in transplanting the entire pancreas?**

Drainage of the pancreatic duct.

☐☐ **What is the most common approach to pancreatic duct drainage?**

Bladder drainage (75%).

☐☐ **T/F: By the time glucose abnormalities are seen after pancreas transplantation, rejection is too far advanced for reversal.**

True.

☐☐ **What is the survival of pancreatic grafts at 36 months?**

Greater than 60%.

☐☐ **What are cluster transplants?**

Transplantation of multiple organs at the same time (i.e., liver-duodenum-pancreas, liver-stomach-duodenum and liver-intestine en bloc).

☐☐ **T/F: There is a high incidence of GVH disease with small bowel transplantation.**

False, despite the large amount of lymphoid tissue within the small bowel.

☐☐ **T/F: Liver transplants are usually orthotopic.**

True.

❑❑ **What is the most common liver disease for which liver transplantation is required?**

Chronic active hepatitis.

❑❑ **T/F: Alcoholism is a contraindication to liver transplantation.**

True, unless the patient has abstained from alcohol for at least two years.

❑❑ **What are the contraindications to liver transplantation?**

Uncontrollable infection, widespread malignancy, concurrent disease (e.g., myocardial infarction) and high risk for recurrent disease in the graft.

❑❑ **What is involved in the initial work-up of potential recipients of liver grafts?**

History and physical, chest x-ray, ECG, serum electrolytes and a fasting blood glucose.

❑❑ **T/F: HLA matching is required for liver transplantation.**

False.

❑❑ **T/F: Smokers must stop smoking prior to liver transplantation.**

True.

❑❑ **What are the most important systems to optimize prior to liver transplantation?**

Nutrition and pulmonary.

❑❑ **T/F: Prophylactic antibiotics are part of the immediate pretransplant protocol.**

True.

❑❑ **What is the most common approach for an orthotopic liver graft?**

A transverse abdominal incision.

❑❑ **What are the preferred immunosuppressive agents in liver transplant patients who have satisfactory renal function?**

Cyclosporine and prednisone.

❑❑ **T/F: Acute tubular necrosis (ATN) is common in the immediate postoperative period.**

True.

❑❑ **When is a radionuclide excretory cholangiogram performed after liver transplantation?**

On postoperative day 3 and then at weekly intervals.

❑❑ **How is liver rejection differentiated from ischemia, viral infection and cholangitis?**

Percutaneous liver biopsy.

❑❑ **What is the most serious complication of liver transplantation?**

Primary nonfunction of the graft.

❏❏ **What is the first indication of primary nonfunction of a liver graft?**

Factor V levels fail to return to normal.

❏❏ **What are the contraindications to cardiac transplantation?**

Systemic disease, irreversible renal/hepatic insufficiency, neoplasia, high/fixed pulmonary vascular resistance and active infection.

❏❏ **What are the most common diseases for which cardiac transplantation is required?**

Congestive cardiomyopathies.

❏❏ **What is the end-stage pathology of cardiomyopathy?**

Dilated cardiac chambers, myocardial degeneration and fibrosis.

❏❏ **T/F: Men receive cardiac transplant much more often than women.**

True.

❏❏ **T/F: ABO compatibility is not a major factor in cardiac transplantation.**

False.

❏❏ **Where is the recipient aorta cross-clamped prior to cardiac transplantation?**

Just proximal to the innominate artery.

❏❏ **What is the most common regimen of immunosuppression following cardiac transplantation?**

Triple therapy with oral cyclosporine, AZ and prednisone.

❏❏ **What drugs are used for induction therapy for patients at high risk of cyclosporine nephrotoxicity?**

Cytolytic agents (OKT3, ATG and ALG).

❏❏ **How is rejection monitored in cardiac graft recipients?**

Weekly right ventricular endomyocardial biopsies.

❏❏ **What hemodynamics are associated with cardiac rejection?**

A low cardiac output, low mixed venous oxygen saturation and elevated right atrial or wedge pressure.

❏❏ **What biopsy findings suggest Grade 3A cardiac rejection?**

Multiple infiltrates with myocyte necrosis.

❏❏ **What signs and symptoms are associated with cardiac rejection?**

Malaise, fatigue, dyspnea/orthopnea, tachycardia, a ventricular gallop, rales and edema.

❏❏ **What is the 5-year survival rate following cardiac transplantation?**

70%.

❑❑ **What are the most common cardiac causes of early mortality in cardiac transplant patients?**

Poor donor selection, poor donor preservation and prohibitive pulmonary hypertension.

❑❑ **What is the major cause of mortality in the first year following cardiac transplantation?**

Infection.

❑❑ **T/F: Graft coronary disease is often treated with coronary artery bypass graft (CABG) or angioplasty.**

False.

❑❑ **What is the standard approach to patients requiring transplantation of both lungs?**

Bilateral single-lung transplantation.

❑❑ **What are the characteristics of end-stage pulmonary disease?**

Respiratory insufficiency and cor pulmonale.

❑❑ **What are the indications for single-lung transplantation?**

Emphysema, pulmonary fibrosis and pulmonary hypertension.

❑❑ **What are the donor pulmonary requirements for lung transplantation?**

Normal gas exchange, a clear chest x-ray and clean tracheobronchial secretions.

❑❑ **T/F: Lungs deteriorate more quickly than any other solid organ in patients with brain death.**

True.

❑❑ **What percentage of heart donors are also suitable lung donors?**

30%.

❑❑ **How is the predicted vital capacity derived?**

From a nomogram based on the patient's height, age and gender.

❑❑ **T/F: Size-matching is more important in double-lung than single-lung transplantation.**

True.

❑❑ **What is the preferred surgical approach for single-lung transplantation?**

A posterolateral thoracotomy.

❑❑ **What are the key technical factors in heart-lung transplantation?**

Good hemostasis of the middle mediastinum and protection of both phrenic nerves, both vagus nerves and the recurrent nerve.

❑❑ **What is Class A lung rejection?**

Acute rejection.

❏❏ **What biopsy findings are associated with chronic vascular rejection?**

Dense infiltrates extending into the alveoli.

❏❏ **What is the 30-day mortality rate for patients with heart-lung transplants?**

20%.

❏❏ **What are the absolute contraindications to renal transplantation?**

Active infection or malignancy that cannot be brought under control.

❏❏ **What is required in the evaluation of the urinary tract prior to renal transplantation?**

A voiding cystogram.

❏❏ **How often does 100% HLA matching occur in siblings?**

25%. (Simple genetics!!)

❏❏ **What type of rejection occurs in renal transplantation when the recipient has preformed antibodies against the donor?**

Hyperacute.

❏❏ **T/F: All patients require dialysis prior to renal transplantation.**

False. However, most do.

❏❏ **T/F: Sibling renal grafts that are poorly matched are more successful than well-matched cadaver grafts.**

True.

❏❏ **What are the advantages of living-related kidney donors?**

The delay between renal failure and rehabilitation is shorter, post-transplant renal function is usually immediate and there are fewer rejection episodes.

❏❏ **What is the definition of brain death?**

Irreversible cessation of all functions of the brain and brainstem.

❏❏ **What are the clinical criteria for brain death?**

1. Fixed and dilated pupils.
2. Absent reflexes.
3. Unresponsive to external stimuli.
4. Inability to maintain vital functions (e.g., respiration, heartbeat and blood pressure) without artificial assistance.

❏❏ **What is the standard immunosuppressive management following renal transplantation?**

Cyclosporine, AZ and prednisone.

❏❏ **What are the best assays of renal function?**

BUN, serum creatinine and creatinine clearance.

❏❏ **How is the diagnosis of ATN made following renal transplantation?**

By exclusion of all other causes of renal failure.

AMPUTATION PEARLS

Any fool can cut off a leg —— it takes a surgeon to save one . . .
George C. Ross

❏❏ **What are the general indications for amputation?**

Extensive trauma, tumor, extensive infection and peripheral vascular disease (PVD).

❏❏ **What is the most common indication for amputation in the United States?**

PVD.

❏❏ **What determines the healing ability of an amputation stump?**

The adequacy of the nutritional blood flow to the skin.

❏❏ **What are the main categories of PVD for which amputation is performed?**

Arteriosclerosis obliterans, arteriosclerosis obliterans with diabetes, thromboangiitis obliterans and miscellaneous (e.g., embolic occlusion and aneurysm).

❏❏ **T/F: Patients with an above the knee amputation (AKA) expend twice the energy to ambulate as those with a below the knee amputation (BKA).**

True.

❏❏ **What is involved in proper postoperative care following amputation?**

Compression dressings followed by elastic dressings to avoid stump edema, splinting of the stump, exercise, proper positioning and early rehabilitation.

❏❏ **What is the operative mortality for amputation performed for trauma, isolated tumor or infection?**

Less than 0.3%.

❏❏ **In what type of amputation are the transected muscles attached to bone by suturing through drill holes?**

Myodesis.

❏❏ **What is the oldest type of amputation in which the tissues are cut in a circular manner?**

The open (guillotine) amputation.

❏❏ **What is the most common indication for lower extremity amputation?**

Ischemia.

❏❏ **T/F: The mortality rate for amputations is higher for more proximal amputations than for distal ones.**

True.

❏❏ **What is the most common intraoperative cause of death during an amputation procedure?**

Cardiac complications.

❏❏ **T/F: There is a direct relationship between the healing of a transmetatarsala amputation and the presence of a palpable popliteal pulse.**

True.

❏❏ **T/F: The tibialis anterior tendon is preserved in a midtarsal amputation.**

True.

❏❏ **What is the procedure of choice when most of the foot has been destroyed?**

A Syme amputation.

❏❏ **T/F: A BKA stump that is too short for a prosthesis is superior to an AKA.**

True.

❏❏ **T/F: Healing of a BKA is decreased by the absence of a popliteal pulse.**

False.

❏❏ **What are the advantages of knee disarticulation?**

It maintains the epiphysis in children, provides maximal length and provides good weight-bearing ability.

❏❏ **What are the absolute indications for an AKA?**

Extension of gangrene to a level that would prevent a BKA and rigor of the calf muscles.

❏❏ **T/F: The mortality rate for AKAs is higher than for any other level of lower extremity amputation.**

True.

❏❏ **T/F: Hemipelvectomy precludes childbirth.**

False.

❏❏ **What are the functions of an artificial limb?**

Gait symmetry, low energy requirement for walking and cosmesis.

❏❏ **What are the requirements for a lower extremity prosthesis?**

A socket to interface with the residual limb (stump) and a suspension device.

❏❏ **What is the most common type of prosthetic socket for a BK amputee?**

The patellar-tendon-bearing type (PTB).

☐☐ **T/F: A BKA is easier to perform than an AKA.**

False.

BIBLIOGRAPHY

BOOKS/ARTICLES

Adler, JN & Plantz, SH. *Emergency Medicine Pearls of Wisdom.* 4th ed. Watertown: Mt. Auburn Press; 1997.

Advanced Cardiac Life Support. Dallas: American Heart Association; 1996.

Advanced Trauma Life Support. Chicago: American College of Surgeons; 1990.

Albert, DM. *Clinical Practice Principles and Practice of Ophthalmology.* Vol. 2. Philadelphia: W.B. Saunders Company; 1994.

American Academy of Ophthalmology. Basic and Clinical Science Course. Vol. 12; 1996-1997.

American Sleep Disorders Association: ICSD--International Classifiaction of Sleep Disorders: diagnostic and Coding Manual, revised. Diagnostic Classification Steering Committee, Thorpy M (chair). Rochester: 1997.

Anderson, JE. *Grant's Atlas of Anatomy.* 8th ed. Baltimore: Williams & Wilkins; 1983.

Auerbach, PS. *Management of Wilderness and Environmental Emergencies.* 2nd ed. St. Louis: CV Mosby Company; 1989.

Bakerman, S. *ABCs of Interpretive Laboratory Data.* 2nd ed. Greenville: Interpretive Laboratory Data, Inc.; 1984.

Barkin, RM. *Emergency Pediatrics.* 3rd ed. St. Louis: CV Mosby Company; 1990.

Berkow, R. *The Merck Manual.* 15th ed. Rahway: Merck Sharp & Dohme Research Laboratories; 1987.

Bork, K. *Diagnosis and Treatment of Common Skin Diseases.* Philadelphia: WB Saunders Company; 1988.

Bradley, WG. *Neurology In Clinical Practice.* Newtown: Butterworth-Heineman; 1996.

Bryson, PD. *Comprehensive Review in Toxicology.* 2nd ed. Aspen Publishers, Inc.; 1989

Bullock, R. *Guidelines for the Management of Severe Head Injury.* New York: Brain Trauma Foundation; 1995.

Cahill, BC. *Clinics in Chest Medicine; 1994.*

Civetta, JM. *Critical Care.* 3rd ed. New York: Lippencott-Raven Publishers; 1997.

Cullom, RD Jr. *The Wills Eye Manual: Office and Emergency Room Diagnosis and Treatment of Eye Disease.* 2nd ed. Philadelphia: JB Lippencott Co.; 1994.

Dambro, MR. *Griffith's 5 Minute Clinical Consult.* Williams and Wilkins; 1996.

DeGowin, EL. *Bedside Diagnostic Examination.* 4th ed. New York: Macmillan Publishing Co. Inc; 1981.

Diagnostic and Treatment Guidelines on Domestic Violence, AMA Publication.

Diagnostic and Treatment Guidelines on Sexual Assault, AMA Publication.

Firearm Violence: Community Diagnosis and Treatment, Publication and slide show of Physicians for Social Responsibility

Fitzpatrick, TB. *Color Atlas and Synopsis of Clinical Dermatology.* New York: McGraw-Hill Publishing Company; 1990.

Flomenbaum, Neal. *Emergency Diagnostic Testing.* 2nd ed. St. Louis: Mosby-Year Book, Inc.; 1995.

Gooch, CL. *Neuroimmunology for Clinicians.* Rolak & Harati; 1996.

Harris, JH. *The Radiology of Emergency Medicine.* 2nd ed. Baltimore: Williams and Wilkins; 1981.

Harrison, TR. *Principles of Internal Medicine.* 11th ed. New York: McGraw-Hill Book Company; 1987.

Harwood-Nuss, A. *The Clinical Practice of Emergency Medicine.* Philadelphia: JB Lippincott Company; 1991.

Harwood-Nuss, A. *The Clinical Practice of Emergency Medicine.* 2nd ed. Philadelphia: JB Lippincott Company; 1996.

Holland, JF. *Cancer Medicine.* 4th ed. Baltimore: Williams & Wilkins; 1997.

Hoppenfeld, S. *Physical Examination of the Spine and Extremities.* Norwalk: Appleton-Century-Crofts; 1976.

Kaplan, HI. *Comprehensive Textbook pf Psychiatry/VI.* 6th ed. Vol. 1.

Koenig, K. *Clinical Emergency Medicine.* New York: McGraw-Hill Inc.; 1996.

Kryger, M. *Principles and Practice of Sleep Medicine.* 2nd ed. Philadelphia: W.B. Saunders Company, 1994.

Leaverton, PE. *A Review of Biostatistics.* 3rd ed. Boston: Little Brown and Company; 1986.

Marriott, HJL. *Practical Electrocardiography.* 7th ed. Baltimore: Williams and Wilkins; 1983.

Moore, KL. *Clinically Oriented Anatomy.* Baltimore: Williams & Wilkins; 1982.

Narayan, RK. *Neurotrauma.* New York: McGraw-Hill Inc.; 1996.

Nelson, W.E. *Textbook of Pediatrics.* Philadelphia: W.B. Saunders Company, 1984.

Pepose, JS. *Ocular Infection and Immunity.* St. Louis: Mosby; 1995.
Perkins, ES. *An Atlas of Diseases of the Eye.* 3rd ed. London: Churchill Livingstone; 1986.

Physicians' Desk Reference. 50th ed. Oradell: Medical Economics Company Inc.; 1996.

Plantz, SH. *Emergency Medicine PreTest, Self-Assessment and Review,* McGraw-Hill Inc.; 1990.

Plantz, SH. *Emergency Medicine.* Baltimore: Wiiliams & Wilkins; 1998.

Rivers, CS. *Preparing for the Written Board Examination in Emergency Medicine.* Milford: Emergency Medicine Educational Enterprises, Inc.; 1992.

Robbins, SL. *Pathologic Basis of Disease*. 3rd ed. Philadelphia: WB Saunders Company; 1984.

Roland, L. *Merritt's Textbook of Neurology*. Williams & Wilkins; 1995.

Rosen, P. *Emergency Medicine Concepts and Clinical Practice*. 3rd ed. St. Louis: Mosby Year Book; 1992.

Rowe, RC. *The Harriet Lane Handbook*. 11th ed. Chicago: Year Book Medical Publishers, Inc.; 1987.

Sabiston, DC, Jr. *Textbook of Surgery*. 14th ed. Philadelphia: WB Saunders Company; 1994.

Schwartz, SI. *Principles of Surgery*. 6th ed. Philadelphia: McGraw-Hill Inc.; 1994.

Shapiro, BA. *Clinical Application of Blood Gases*. 5th ed. St. Louis: Mosby-Year Book, Inc.; 1994.

Simon, RR. *Emergency Orthopedics The Extremities*. 2nd ed. Norwalk: Appleton & Lange; 1987.

Simon, RR. *Emergency Procedures and Techniques*. 2nd ed. Baltimore: Williams and Wilkins; 1987.

Slaby, F. *Radiographic Anatomy*. New York: John Wiley & Sons; 1990.

Squire, LF. *Fundamentals of Radiology*. 3rd ed. Cambridge: Harvard University Press; 1982.

Stedman, TL. *Illustrated Stedman's Medical Dictionary*. 24th ed. Baltimore: Williams & Wilkins; 1982.

Stewart, CE. *Environmental Emergencies*. Baltimore: Williams and Wilkins; 1990.

Textbook of Pediatric Advanced Life Support. Dallas: American Heart Association; 1988.

The Hand Examination and Diagnosis. 2nd ed. London: Churchill Livingstone; 1983.

The Hand Primary Care of Common Problems. 2nd ed. London: Churchill Livingstone; 1990.

The Physician's Guide to Domestic Violence. Salber and Taliaferro, Volcano Press; 1995

Tintinalli, JE. *Emergency Medicine A Comprehensive Study Guide*. 4th ed. New York: McGraw-Hill, Inc.; 1996.

Tsang T, Demby AM. Penile fracture with urethral injury. *Journal of Urology*. 1992; vol. 147: 466-468.

Weinberg, S. *Color Atlas of Pediatric Dermatology*. 2nd ed. New York: McGraw-Hill Inc.; 1990.

Weiner, HL. *Neurology for the House Officer*. 4th ed. Baltimore: Williams & Wilkins; 1989.

Wilkins, EW. *Emergency Medicine*. 3rd ed. Baltimore: Williams & Wilkins; 1989.

Wilkins, RH. *Neurosurgery*. New York: McGraw-Hill; 1996.

Wilkinson, CP. *Retinal Detachment*. New York: Mosby; 1997.

Youmans, JR. *Neurological Surgery*. Philadelphia: W.B. Saunders; 1996.

COURSES/CONFERENCES

Eye Diseases and Emergencies. Chicago, IL; 1991.

ENT Diseases and Emergencies. Chicago, IL; 1991.

CRIT Course. Springfield, MA; 1992.

Interactive Board Review. Boca Raton, FL; 1992.

EMS: A Trauma Update. Sponsored by Boston Medflight, Plymouth, MA; 1994.

Selected Topics in Emergency Medicine. Sponsored by MGH and Brigham and Women's Hospitals and Harvard Medical School, Boston, MA; 1995, 1996.

Emergency Medicine: Update and Current Practice. Sponsored by MGH ED and Harvard Medical School, Boston, MA; 1994, 1995, 1996.

Update on New Techniques and Review of Established Principles of Management of Cerebrovascular Emergencies. Sponsored by MGH Brain Aneurysm/AVM Center, Neurointensive Care Unit and ED, Boston, MA; 1996.

www.ingramcontent.com/pod-product-compliance
Ingram Content Group UK Ltd.
Pitfield, Milton Keynes, MK11 3LW, UK
UKHW051300180426
11947UKWH00020B/1829